The Ultimate Castor Oil Bible

A Complete Guide to Natural Beauty, Hair Growth, and Joint Pain Relief

Catalina R. Brooks

Table of Contents

Dedication

To my mother, who taught me the gift of natural remedies and the love of taking care of oneself, your wisdom and love continue to inspire me daily. This book honours your nurturing spirit and the knowledge you've passed down through generations.

Acknowledgments

Writing The Ultimate Castor Oil Bible has been a journey of self-discovery, learning, and significant growth. I am eternally grateful to those who have stood by me.

First and foremost, I would like to thank my family for their endless support and encouragement, my husband for being there and patiently listening to my innumerable discussions about castor oil, and for the feedback that is always so valued- to him, my greatest champion. And then my children constantly remind me of the beauty and wonder in this world. Love sustains me and keeps me grounded yet inspired.

A special thank you to the innumerable experts, herbalists, and wellness professionals who taught me. Your decades-long commitment to natural health and healing has influenced this book on many levels.

Last but not least, to my readers, thanks for your interest in and commitment to natural remedies. This book will equip you with the incredible benefits of castor oil for your health and well-being. Your journey toward natural beauty and healing inspires me, and I am honoured to participate in this process.

With appreciation,

Catalina R. Brooks

Introduction

Welcome to the Ultimate Castor Oil Bible

Castor oil is considered versatile and instrumental in health and cosmetic therapies and has been regarded so for many centuries. This thick, light oil expressed from the seeds of the castor plant, Ricinus communis, has crossed cultures, geographies, and centuries to earn its reputation as a natural elixir for wellness and healing. Presently, castor oil is finding favor with consumers in their quests for more natural and sustainable options against manufactured products. The history of castor oil, how unique it is in the market today, and what science behind incredible works would be introduced here.

Overview of Castor Oil's Benefits

Castor oil is derived from the seeds of a plant called Ricinus communis and has been a welcome remedy for its magical touch in healing for many years. Known to be multipurpose, this thick, viscous oil finds its way into various health and beauty routines across cultures and generations. Castor oil presents a natural, effective remedy for chronic pain relief, improving natural beauty or general well-being. The succeeding section illustrates the significant benefits of castor oil that make it indispensable in your wellness toolkit.

Skin Care: A Natural Moisturizer and Healer

Castor oil is an excellent emollient, thus capable of reaching the skin to hydrate and feed it from the inside. Its high concentration of ricinoleic acid makes it a superb moisturizer, particularly for dry, flaky, and damaged skin. Besides its moisturizing properties, castor oil is also used as a remedy for many skin problems, including acne, eczema, and psoriasis, due to its anti-inflammatory and antimicrobial properties.

- **Hydration and Moisturization:** Castor oil seals it, preventing water loss and keeping your skin supple and smooth.
- **Anti-Aging:** Due to the stimulation of collagen production, it reduces the appearance of fine lines and wrinkles, hence leaving your skin looking younger and brighter.
- **Healing Wounds and Scars:** Castor oil stimulates quicker wound healing due to its anti-inflammatory effects and stimulating tissue regeneration; hence, it will help minimize scars and stretch marks.

Hair Care: Promoting Growth and Health

Castor oil has been used for ages to aid in hair care naturally. More specifically, it is known for stimulating hair growth by strengthening strands and adding shine. Whether you are having problems with hair loss or dandruff or just want to bring out the natural beauty of your hair, castor oil will play a major role.

- **Hair Growth:** Castor oil's beneficial properties stimulate the hair follicles, encouraging the thicker and more robust growth of hair. It is very effective for thinning hair or hair loss.
- **Scalp Health:** Castor oil keeps your scalp healthy because of its anti-fungal and anti-bacterial properties. This reduces dandruff and prevents scalp infections.

- **Conditioning:** Castor oil should be used regularly to moisturize the hair; this makes it less frizzy with split ends and gives it a natural shine.

Joint and Muscle Relief: Easing Pain Naturally

Castor oil's anti-inflammatory properties make it a powerful ally in managing pain associated with arthritis, muscle aches, and joint discomfort. When applied topically, castor oil penetrates deep into tissues, relieving inflammation and pain.

- **Arthritis Relief:** Regularly applying castor oil on inflamed joints will reduce stiffness, increase mobility, and relieve pain.
- **Muscle Relaxation:** Castor oil is an excellent choice for post-exercise recovery. It can be massaged into sore muscles to relieve tension and promote relaxation.
- **Chronic Pain Management:** Castor oil is one such natural alternative to the chemical-laden pain relievers that promise relief from chronic pain disorders like fibromyalgia without any side effects.

Digestive Health: A Gentle Cleanser

Castor oil is traditionally used as a mild laxative to help eliminate constipation and clean the system. Its smooth yet effective action makes it commendable for people who value natural health in digestion.

- **Relieving Constipation:** Castor oil has been traditionally used to induce bowel movements to achieve relief from constipation and ensure regularity.

- **Detoxification:** Castor oil aids in the body's natural detoxification process by helping to eliminate waste, cleanse the liver, and purify the intestines.
- **Gut Health:** The anti-inflammatory properties of castor oil would soothe the digestive tract and mitigate the symptoms of IBS and other digestive disorders.

Immune System Support: Boosting Natural Defenses

Castor oil's ability to stimulate the lymphatic system makes it an exceptional tool for enhancing immune function. The lymphatic system is pivotal in the body's defense against infection, and castor oil helps keep this system at an optimal status.

- **Lymphatic Drainage:** The application of castor oil packs encourages lymphatic drainage, hence removing toxins that reduce the activity of the lymphatic system.
- **Anti-Inflammatory Effects:** Castor oil also prevents inflammation, increasing the immune system's capacity to fight infection and maintain health in general.
- **Overall Wellness:** By topical application or ingesting castor oil repeatedly, one is enhancing one's immune system to become strong enough to prevent illness from taking over one's body quickly.

Why This Book is Your Go-To Resource

Finding a reliable and comprehensive guide can sometimes be annoyingly hard in a world swollen with information. *The Ultimate Castor Oil Bible* is designed to be a trusted resource that presents everything you could hope to know about this incredible oil. Whether you are advanced in natural health or just exploring this wonderful world of holistic wellness, this book is filled with valuable insights and practical advice that can be applied in daily life.

Comprehensive and Research-Based Information

This book combines traditional knowledge gained over many centuries with modern scientific research, enabling you to learn about the benefits of castor oil on many levels. You will go through detailed descriptions with studies and experts supporting this notion, ensuring the information you get is proper and timely.

Practical Applications for Everyday Life

The Ultimate Castor Oil Bible is not some theory; this book teaches step-by-step, easy-to-follow instructions on infusing castor oil into your life. From do-it-yourself beauty recipes to treatments for instant pain relief, you'll find each chapter filled with actionable tips you can immediately implement.

Tailored for Your Specific Needs

If you want to learn about using castor oil for natural beauty enhancement, relieving chronic pain, or simply for general health enhancement, this book is structured to meet your needs. Each chapter of this book has been devoted to a particular aspect of the benefits derivable from castor oil; hence, you will efficiently and quickly get to the information that interests you the most.

User-Friendly Layout and Accessible Language

Written in accessible, jargon-free language, this book is for anyone, regardless of background. Its easy-to-use format, clear step-by-step instructions, quick-reference tables, and lavish illustrations make it easy to use and navigate, whether you read from cover to cover or dip in for advice on a particular subject.

Expert Tips and Personal Insights

The author draws on years of experience and expertise, making the book often comprising personal insights and expert tips. These little nuggets will enable you to avoid common pitfalls and ensure you derive the maximum from your castor oil regimen.

How to Use This Book for Maximum Benefit

Approaching this book as both a guide and a practical tool helps to approach each of the many uses and the power of castor oil. Here is how one can get the most from *The Ultimate Castor Oil Bible*:

Start with the Basics

If you are new to castor oil, read the introductory chapters about its history, properties, and general benefits. This will set a perfect foundation and help you appreciate why castor oil works so well in various health and beauty applications.

Identify Your Primary Goals

You say what you want to achieve using castor oil- perfect skin, hair growth, or pain relief from body detoxification.

Once you have identified this, you can be keenly interested in those chapters that relate to your needs.

Follow the Step-by-Step Guides

Each chapter explains how castor oil should be used for a particular purpose. Observe the recommended dosages, methods of application, and the frequency of application with attention to the guides. The undemanding reading of the step-by-step format makes it easier to follow these practices in your daily routine.

Customize Your Routine

Castor oil is versatile, and this book will encourage you to try different recipes and methods to find your perfect match. Take all the DIY recipes and suggestions in this book as a starting point, and do not hesitate to make changes if that works for you or fits your particular needs.

Track Your Progress

You can easily record how your body responds to castor oil treatment with a diary or some notes. Note skin, hair, digestion, or other aches and pains that may improve, making adjustments as needed. By doing this, you can tailor your routine to fit your needs and ensure you're gaining the full benefit from your castor oil experience.

Use the Appendices for Quick Reference

Appendixes at the end contain quick reference guides on common concerns, DIY recipes, storage, and further resources. Refer to them whenever you need a quick answer or information beyond the normal realms.

Share Your Knowledge

Share the wonders of castor oil with others, either friends or family, as you learn more about it. Though this book is for anyone's use, besides that, your own experiences can also encourage others to start examining for themselves the many uses and benefits that come from castor oil.

The Ultimate Castor Oil Bible is way more than a simple book; it is an informative roadmap through how one can exploit, to its fullness, one of nature's most potent oils. Through this book, by learning the science behind castor oil and instituting some practical advice, you'll realize long-lasting changes in health, beauty, and overall well-being. Whether you have particular needs or wish to enhance your current natural wellness regimen, this book will be your ultimate handbook for castor oil. Welcome to the path to a healthier, livelier you with the help of this valuable guidebook.

Part 1: Castor Oil for Natural Beauty

Chapter 1:
The Beauty Elixir-How Castor Oil Transforms Your Skin

Castor oil is that one beauty secret which everyone knows, yet it has umpteen benefits for your skin-from superficial to deep tissue problems. Castor oil, as strong natural medicine, could be applied to stubborn marks to make them heal, to wrinkles to reduce their appearance, and to dry areas to hydrate them. This chapter will expound on the many ways that castor oil can enrich your skincare and turn lifeless, problematic skin into glowing, healthy-looking skin.

History of Castor Oil: From Ancient Uses to Modern Discoveries

Castor oil is believed to have a very ancient history, back to ancient Egypt, where it had a liking for its medication and cosmetic benefits. Castor oil was traced in the tombs of Egyptian kings and is believed to have been used as an embalming agent, skin moisturizer, and a source of light fuel. According to history, Cleopatra used castor oil to whiten her eyes, thus revealing the oil's attachment to beauty since time immemorial.

Castor oil was utilized in Ayurveda, one of the most ancient holistic treatments of India. The Ayurvedic practitioners used castor oil for anti-inflammatory, laxative, and pain-relieving effects. It was given to treat stomach problems, joint aches, and skin diseases, making its standing as a versatile medicine.

Castor oil continued to grow in popularity, and during the Roman Empire, the drug became one of the highly used laxatives, as well as for treating a wide range of diseases, such as skin disorders and arthritis. During medieval Europe, the oil was used for treating wounds and skin irritations. The versatility of castor oil was important in making this an integral part of life across cultures, particularly for those interested in natural and effective therapies in times before modern medicine.

With the advent of modern science, castor oil became ever more in demand within the pharmaceutical industry. In the 18th and 19th centuries, castor oil was freely available in both Europe and America, where it was used as a general remedy for stomach ailments, coughs, and colds. Further on, several investigations were carried out on the strange chemical composition of castor oil and its new uses as an aggressive oil.

Today, the oil is better known not only for its conventional medical applications but also for effectiveness in cosmetics, hair care, and even industrial products such as lubricants and biofuel. In recent times, the various benefits offered by castor oil were sought after once again and therefore brought it into the limelight as one of the popular remedies for natural beauty and health.

One of the distinguishing features of castor oil is the way it is processed; this largely influences its quality, effectiveness, and even safety. The cold-pressed form of castor oil is considered to be the very best quality. A mechanical procedure, cold-pressing entails crushing castor seeds to extract oil content in the absence of heat. Without heating, the oil retains its full nutrient profile, including enzymes and other beneficial compounds, which makes cold-pressed castor oil perfect even for internal and external use.

Cold-pressed castor oil is often free from additives and chemicals and maintains its natural potency. This is in contrast to more industrially prepared castor oils, which use heat and chemical solvents in the process of extraction. One such solvent is hexane, used in cheaper oils for the purpose of increasing production, although this may diminish the quality of the oil. Hexane-free castor oil means that hazardous chemicals are not added during the processing of such oil, making it much safer for customers to use, intended for personal care or even for consumption.

Another available choice for most customers in the market, aside from cold-pressed and hexane-free, is organic castor oil. Organic certification assures that at the time of farming, the castor plants did not involve the use of synthetic pesticides, fertilizers, or GMOs. This not only keeps the product cleaner but also supports more ecologically friendly modes of farming. Organic castor oil is particularly popular among those who are apprehensive about what they apply to their skin or consume and who prefer greens, cruelty-free products.

Another very popular variant is the Jamaican black castor oil, which is extracted in a totally different way than conventional castor oil. During this process, the seeds get roasted before pressing, yielding oil that is darker and thicker, packing more nutrients within. This category of oil is, in particular, in high demand for stimulating hair growth and scalp care; hence, it is usually sought after by people who want to give new life to their balding or thinning hair.

Cold-pressed, hexane-free, and organic castor oil are the highest standards in natural oil production, meeting the rising demand for high-over-quality, chemical-free wellness products. Whether for cosmetic, hair care, or health cures, these variants assure the inherent purity of castor oil and deliver optimum benefits to their consumers.

Why Castor Oil Works: Unraveling the Science Behind Nature's Miracle Oil

Castor oil owes its rich list of benefits to its peculiar chemical composition, where one single fatty acid called ricinoleic acid predominates, making up more than 90% of its composition. In fact, it is due to this very factor-ricinoleic acid-that sets castor oil apart from other oils and possesses formidable anti-inflammatory, antibacterial, and moisturizing characteristics. These qualities enable castor oil to treat different skin diseases, pain relief, and the initiation of hair growth.

Administered topically, ricinoleic acid penetrates deep into the skin, giving moisture and reducing inflammation. It has made castor oil an effective natural remedy for diseases like eczema, psoriasis, and dry skin. Its moisturizing effect further enhances the natural barrier function of the skin, reduces irritation, and accelerates the healing process.

The thick viscosity and nutrient-rich profile of castor oil confer a number of benefits related to hair care: scalp conditioning, dandruff fighting, and hardening hair follicles. Ricinoleic acid provides efficient stimulating of blood flow to the scalp to encourage hair growth. In fact, castor oil has been a very popular solution among people suffering from thinning hair or hair loss over the past little while.

The anti-inflammatory properties of Castor oil, along with increased blood flow to affected areas, are responsible for therapeutic analgesic effects. Research has verified that the use of castor oil packs or massage using this oil as an active remedy for arthritis, muscular pains, and joint pains. It increases circulation, hence is good for small injuries and edema reduction.

Castor oil is well known for its natural laxative action taken internally. The ricinoleic acid, on ingestion, acts to cause spasms in the intestinal muscles, promoting bowel movement and hence relieving constipation. Castor oil does not become as harsh on the body like other synthetic laxatives and at times can be used to relieve stomach ache; however, it should be taken accordingly to avoid any side effects.

Furthermore, it is confirmed that castor oil stimulates the lymphatic system; hence, it helps to cleanse and increase the immunological function of the human body. Therefore, this explains its use in some holistic therapies aimed at making enriching general health through stimulation of the natural mechanisms for self-healing set by the body.

In combination with other important fatty acids, ricinoleic acid forms the base, making castor oil one of the most potent therapies which Mother Nature has to offer. Whether taken for beauty or health purposes, the scientifically explained advantages of castor oil make for a big argument to its continuing use as a natural, holistic remedy.

Hydrating and Smoothing: Castor Oil for Radiant Skin

Because castor oil is high in fatty acids, mainly ricinoleic acid, it is fundamentally a very strong moisturizer. In other words, due to the particular fatty acid responsible for granting castor oil its properties, it completely penetrates into the skin, seals moisture, and hydrates all day long. Its thick texture protects your skin from environmental aggressors like pollution and bad weather conditions, acting like a shield to block water loss from taking place.

Deep Hydration: Castor oil deeply enters the skin layers, hence fighting dryness from within and leaving the skin smooth and supple. Anyone with Any Skin Type Can Apply Castor Oil: Though highly good for dry and sensitive skin, oily or combination skin types can also use it because it does not clog pores due to its non-comedogenic properties.

Smoothening of skin: Castor oil, if used on a regular basis, will leave your skin much smoother, supple, and healthy-looking overall.

You could have fully replenished, radiant skin without using any harmful or synthetic chemicals if you just use castor oil as part of your moisturizing routine or even just at night.

Castor Oil for Reducing Wrinkles and Fine Lines as an Anti-Aging Solution

Among all the cosmetic benefits that castor oil possesses, its action against signs of aging remains in high demand. Rich in antioxidants and fatty acids, castor oil acts gently to give a natural solution to saggy skin, fine lines, and wrinkles.

Boosts Collagen synthesis: Collagen and elastin are two essential proteins that keep the skin elastic and firm. Castor oil helps in increasing the synthesis of these proteins. The skin will be young and plump due to the increase in collagen synthesis, which might reduce the fine lines and wrinkles over time.

Smoothing Wrinkles: Vitamin E, along with other antioxidants in castor oil, is useful in fighting against free radicals that accelerate the aging process. It works to neutralize the free radicals to avoid new wrinkles.

Non-Invasive Approach: Unlike chemical-based anti-aging treatments that can be hazardous even to the extent of irritation and other adverse effects, castor oil is a non-toxic natural solution to problems related to aging.

Castor oil is an excellent anti-aging for people seeking a natural alternative to expensive lotions and procedures involving invasion. Anyone using this regularly can be assured of firmer and smoother skin.

Natural Remedies for Blemishes and Acne

Castor oil, due to its anti-bacterial and anti-inflammatory nature, is a great treatment for acne, though generally misjudged because other oils tend to clog pores and worsen the condition. It therefore comes in handy for those seeking all-natural solutions to traditional treatments for acne.

Antibacterial Properties: Ricinoleic acid has strong antibacterial properties to fight off the bacteria Propionibacterium acnes responsible for causing an outbreak of acne.

Reduces Inflammation: The anti-inflammatory properties of castor oil reduce swelling and redness from acne. It soothes irritated skin without the harmful side effects of chemical-based treatments for acne.

Skin Oil Balance: Castor oil regulates skin oil production-much unlike most acne drugs, which dry out the face completely. By keeping the skin moist, it regulates excess oil through controlled sebum, hence reducing breakouts.

This way, your skin is cleaner and healthier without the risk of dryness or irritation that often comes with using over-the-counter treatments for acne. Castor oil works great, both as a natural cleanser for acne, which you can use on a regular basis, and as a skin treatment to help fight against breakouts of the skin.

How to Use Castor Oil for Treating Stretch Marks

Stretch marks are the concern of many people, and they mostly occur as a result of sudden skin stretching because of changes in body weight or pregnancy. Castor oil, due to its deep nourishment and skin elasticity enhancement, is effective in preventing stretch marks and reducing their visibility.

Improves Skin Elasticity: Castor oil stimulates collagen, thereby allowing the skin to stretch without breaking down or scarring. This is highly useful during pregnant stages or when one undergoes a rapid increase or decrease in weight.

Prevents New Stretch Marks: As castor oil keeps the skin moisturized and supple, applying it regularly in areas of the body that are prone to stretch marks will prevent new ones from appearing, such as on the belly, thighs, or hips.

Minimizes the Appearance of Stretch Marks: Castor oil nourishes the already injured skin and thus helps rejuvenate it. Castor oil, being thick, can be massaged deep in the skin to help ensure long-term healing.

Castor oil was utilized in skincare routines to help ward off stretch marks naturally and safely, especially during periods of physical transformation. Because of this, castor oil becomes a helpful tool for any person attempting to keep their skin uniformly smooth.

Castor Oil for Nail and Cuticle Care

Care for the nails and cuticles is important not only for strong, healthy nails but also to avoid many problems related to hangnails, dryness of the nail, and fungal infections. Castor oil is one of the most appropriate and natural treatments to nourish cuticles and nails due to its highly nutritious structure and rich texture. It holds a special combination of vitamins, fatty acids, and anti-fungal qualities, making it very effective in maintaining strong nails and healthy, smooth cuticles. This section will discuss the advantages of using castor oil in your beauty regimen for cuticle and nail care, plus some useful tips on how one does it.

Why Castor Oil Works So Well for Cuticle and Nail Care

Effective Moisturizing

Rich in Fatty Acids: Castor oil is rich in ricinoleic acid, an ultra-moisturizing fatty acid penetrating deep into skin and nails. This makes the oil suitable for thick cuticles and dry, brittle nails. Smearing castor oil regularly will keep the nails moisturized, supple, and less apt to split or break.

This softens cuticles; dry, overgrown cuticles create hangnails, among other nail problems. Castor oil's thickness and hydrating properties make cuticles softer and easier to push back and retain when used. It also prevents cuticle problems, aside from making your nails look better.

Stimulates Nail Growth

Rich in ingredients: Castor oil is rich in vital ingredients like Vitamin E, proteins, and minerals that help nourish and encourage nail growth. Regularly massaging castor oil into your nails will stimulate them to grow stronger and faster. The nutritional value of the oil supports the healing of the nails, promoting overall nail health.

Applying castor oil to your cuticles and nails improves blood flow to the nail beds. The increased nutrition delivered to the nails due to improved circulation allows the nails to grow well and become healthy.

Anti-fungal and Anti-bacterial Action

Prevents Infections: Due to its anti-fungal and anti-bacterial properties, castor oil cures and prevents some common types of nail infections, such as paronychia, an infection of the cuticles, among other fungal nail infections. Massaging castor oil will keep the infection-causing germs and all other problems away from your cuticles and nails.

Strengthens and Protects

Prevents Brittleness: Weak and brittle nails are prone to splitting, breaking, and peeling. Your nails will be much stronger because the strengthening action of the castor oil on the nail plate is due to its nourishing properties. Regular application of castor oil can reduce the frequency of nail splitting and breaking.

Protection Against Environmental Damage: Chemicals, water, and cold temperatures are a few of the harsh environmental elements that cuticles and nails are continuously exposed to. It forms a shield around the nails and cuticles against such elements to protect the nails and cuticles and to preserve their integrity. It acts as a shield and disinfects and cleans the nails and cuticles.

How to Use Castor Oil for Nail and Cuticle Care
Daily Nail and Cuticle Moisturizer

Instructions:

- At the end of your day, apply a small amount of castor oil directly to your nails and cuticles.
- Massage the oil into each nail, focusing on the cuticles, for about 2-3 minutes.
- Allow the oil to absorb fully. You can leave it on overnight for deeper moisturization.
- For best results, repeat this process daily to maintain healthy, hydrated nails and cuticles.

Nail Growth Serum

Ingredients:

- 1 tablespoon of castor oil
- 1 tablespoon of almond oil (or jojoba oil)
- 5 drops of vitamin E oil (optional)

Instructions:

- Mix all ingredients in a small glass bottle with a dropper.

- Apply a drop to each nail and cuticle, massaging in gently.
- Use this serum daily, preferably at night, to promote nail growth and strengthen nails.

Cuticle Softening Treatment

Instructions:

- Before your manicure, apply castor oil generously to your cuticles.
- Let the oil sit for 10-15 minutes to soften the cuticles.
- Gently push back your cuticles using a cuticle pusher or an orange stick.
- Wipe away any excess oil with a clean cloth and proceed with your manicure.
- Regular use of this treatment helps to maintain healthy cuticles and prevent hangnails.

Anti-Fungal Nail Treatment

Instructions:

- If you have a fungal infection or are prone to them, apply castor oil directly to the affected nail and surrounding skin.
- Massage the oil into the nail and cuticle area, allowing it to penetrate deeply.
- For enhanced anti-fungal effects, you can add a few drops of tea tree oil to the castor oil before application.

- Repeat this treatment twice daily until the infection clears. Continued use can help prevent future infections.

Overnight Nail Repair Treatment

Instructions:

- For nails that are particularly weak or damaged, apply a thick layer of castor oil to your nails and cuticles before bed.
- Cover your hands with cotton gloves to lock in the moisture and prevent the oil from rubbing off onto your bedding.
- Leave the oil on overnight, allowing it to deeply nourish and repair your nails while you sleep.
- Use this treatment as needed to restore nail strength and health.

DIY Nail and Cuticle Balm

Ingredients:

- 1 tablespoon of castor oil
- 1 tablespoon of shea butter
- 1 tablespoon of beeswax
- A few drops of your favorite essential oil (e.g., lavender, lemon)

Instructions:

- Melt the shea butter and beeswax in a double boiler.
- Stir in the castor oil and essential oil until well combined.

- Pour the mixture into a small container and let it cool and solidify.
- Apply the balm to your nails and cuticles daily to keep them moisturized, protected, and healthy.

Tips for Maximizing Results

- **The secret lies in making it a habit:** only by using castor oil daily, applied to the nail and cuticle care routine, can the best results be achieved. Regular treatment will strengthen and hydrate nails, avoiding common problems.
- **Combine with a healthy diet:** A healthy diet is rich in vitamins and minerals, like zinc and vitamin E, but especially biotin, which is important for nail health. Topical castor oil treatments should be combined with a healthy diet for best results.
- **Avoid Harsh Chemicals:** Use less time around potent chemicals in the house cleaners and nail paint removers. Considering your nails, the best way to avoid damage and keep them healthy is to wear gloves while using the products above.

Apple cider vinegar and castor oil: A powerful natural combination

Two of nature's most powerful and multiapplication treatments are castor oil and apple cider vinegar. Both conventional medicine and alternative health have been significant beneficiaries of these two treatments for a long. While each treatment is powerful on its own, the combination of castor oil with apple cider vinegar has a synergistic action that improves their benefits for various wellness, cosmetic, and health uses. From digestion to detoxification, hair to skincare, the solution comes from this team of talented naturalists. The unique qualities of castor oil and apple cider vinegar will be discussed here, including how to use them daily and their combined advantages.

Understanding the Properties of Castor Oil and Apple Cider Vinegar

Castor Oil

- **Source:** Castor oil is derived from the seeds of the tropical native Ricinus communis plant. Because of its medicinal effects, this plant has been used since time immemorial in several cultures throughout the world.
- **Essential Elements:** Ricinoleic acid is the major active ingredient in castor oil; its content is appropriate for exerting anti-inflammatory, antibacterial, and moisturizing effects. This oil also contains omega-6 and omega-9 fatty acids, vitamin E, and other healthy elements.
- **Uses:** It finds its application as one of the most common nonsynthetic oils for pain treatment, detoxification, maintenance of digestive health, skincare, and hair treatment. This oil is a natural remedy for many conditions because of its thickness and deep skin penetration ability.

Apple Cider Vinegar (ACV)

- **Source:** Apples have to undergo a two-step fermentation process in order for the sugars to be converted to acetic acid, which would constitute the preparation method of vinegar through the use of apple cider. ACV has conventionally been used for many thousands of years as a method of preservation, medicinal use, and cooking.

- **Essential Ingredients:** The main active ingredient of apple cider vinegar is acetic acid, which is responsible for its special taste and smell. ACV also contains vitamins, minerals, enzymes, and friendly bacteria; this is especially true for unfiltered versions, which are said to have the "mother" within them—a combination of yeast and bacteria.

- **Uses:** These mainly include digestion, weight problems, blood sugar regulation, skin care, and hair care. It also has antifungal, antibacterial, and anti-inflammatory actions, among others.

Benefits of Combining Castor Oil and Apple Cider Vinegar

This can be pretty effective since the complementary nature of these two ingredients allows them to enhance their properties upon mixing. The combination has powerful benefits in treating various health and cosmetic problems. Here's how you can apply this mixture:

Skincare Benefits

- **Acne Treatment:** Castor oil's antibacterial action, combined with apple cider vinegar's effectiveness in balancing the skin's pH and reducing inflammation, effectively treats acne and reduces breakouts. The acidity of ACV in exfoliating and unclogging the pores is combined with the healing and moisturizing action of castor oil.

- **Even Skin Tone:** Apple cider vinegar possesses mild acidity, which helps degrade the dead layer of the skin, promoting cell turnover. This helps lighten dark spots and even out your skin tone. The addition of castor oil is moisturizing and nourishing and aids in improving the skin's texture and appearance.
- **Anti-Aging:** The moisturizing effect of castor oil combined with the exfoliating action of ACV can reduce fine lines and wrinkles on your skin. Castor oil deeply moisturizes skin, while apple cider vinegar stimulates collagen production by regenerating it.

Haircare Benefits

- **Scalp Health:** Castor oil and apple cider vinegar have both been associated with scalp health. Castor oil has anti-inflammatory properties that moisturize the scalp to avoid dryness and irritation, while the antimicrobial nature of ACV ensures no dandruff or other scalp conditions occur. Together, they form an environment in harmony with healthy hair growth.
- **Hair Growth:** Castor oil is renowned for its hair growth-enhancing properties since it nourishes and increases blood flow to the scalp. However, when combined with apple cider vinegar's clarifying ability —which can clean the scalp and remove any product buildup—this combination can further enhance hair growth by cleaning the scalp and keeping the follicles adequately fed.

- **Shiny and Smooth Hair:** Apple cider vinegar is generally used as a natural conditioner, smoothing the cuticles of the hair to add shine. Castor oil, on the other hand, contributes its strength and moisturizing content to the strands of hair. When used together, these will lead to hair that is soft and shiny but far stronger and resilient.

Digestive Health Benefits

- **Detoxification:** The detox properties of apple cider vinegar are highly renowned for cleaning the liver and thus supporting digestion. Castor oil is a laxative and will help detoxify by promoting bowel movements and cleaning the digestive tract. In combination, they can support a mild yet effective detox regimen.
- **Digestive Comfort:** Both castor oil and apple cider vinegar soothe digestive disturbances like bloating or indigestion. ACV normalizes stomach acid levels and aids digestion. Anti-inflammatory castor oil eases the digestive tract and allows regularity.

Weight Management

- **Appetite Control:** One of the major properties of apple cider vinegar is that it causes a feeling of fullness in the stomach, thus controlling appetite and reducing calorie intake. Castor oil's detoxification activity will contribute to weight management by ensuring the digestive system works optimally.
- **Improve Metabolism:** Studies have shown that the acetic acid in apple cider vinegar accelerates metabolism and reduces fat accumulation. Combined with castor oil, which furthers detoxification and gut

health, this mixture will aid metabolism for better weight loss.

The Castor Oil and Lemon Detox Drink: A Natural Elixir for Cleansing and Health

Detoxification means clearing the body of waste material, toxins, and other poisonous substances that may build up through poor dieting and environmental exposure, among other lifestyle practices. The human body has some natural detoxification systems, such as the liver, kidneys, and lymphatic system, which are sometimes overloaded. You will be able to nurture these systems and enhance your body's ability for effective self-cleansing by adding a natural detox drink into your daily routine. One of the most potent detox drinks would be the Castor Oil and Lemon Detox Drink, which fuses the energizing and alkalizing attributes of lemon juice with the powerful cleaning features of castor oil. It is a natural potion that supports liver cleaning, increases general health, and promotes digestive health.

Why Castor Oil and Lemon Make a Powerful Detox Duo

Castor Oil: A Potent Natural Cleanser

- **Laxative Properties:** Castor oil is well known to possess strong laxative properties. It facilitates bowel movements to rid the body of toxins within the digestive system. Thus, it becomes an extremely effective way of encouraging regularity and easing constipation—two of the integral parts of any detox program.

- **Anti-Inflammatory and Healing Effects:** The anti-inflammatory nature of ricinoleic acid, the primary active constituent of castor oil, exerts soothing effects on intestinal irritation and prevents inflammation. This can be useful for anyone trying to reduce general inflammation or affected by gut problems.

- **Liver Support:** Traditionally, castor oil is known to aid the functioning of the liver by allowing the free flow of bile, hence increasing the efficiency with which the liver can process toxins and eliminate them from the system. This makes the inclusion of castor oil a necessity in detox drinks for liver cleansing and general detoxing.

Lemon Juice: Nature's Alkalizer and Detoxifier

- **Rich in Vitamin C and Antioxidants:** Lemon juice contains a large amount of vitamin C, which rejuvenates the skin, immune system, and body's refurbishing and repairing abilities. Antioxidants derived from lemon juice are helpful in scavenging free radicals, which can accelerate aging and diseases.

- **Alkalizing Properties:** Although it may be acidic in nature, lemon juice acts like an alkaline agent inside the body after digestion. It minimizes acidity, which creates diseases and inflammation, by balancing the body's pH levels.

- **Digestive Aid:** Lemon juice promotes the production of digestive enzymes responsible for food digestion and absorption. It also has a moderate diuretic effect, which boosts renal performance by facilitating the excretion of toxins via urine.

- **Liver Detoxification:** It helps detoxify the liver by improving its ability to produce bile, a fluid responsible for fat digestion and waste removal from the body. The citric acid present in lemon helps clean the liver, avoiding the deposition of toxins.

Health Benefits of the Castor Oil and Lemon Detox Drink
Enhanced Digestive Health

- **Relieves Constipation:** The castor oil-lemon juice mixture detox drink is effective in reducing constipation due to the laxative properties of castor oil and the digestive advantages of lemon juice. It empties the intestines, automatically reducing bloating and lessening pain since bowel movement is encouraged.
- **Promotes Gut Healing:** Lemon juice assists in better digestion of meals and the absorption of nutrients, while castor oil is anti-inflammatory and soothes the stomach lining. Together, these will reduce the signs and symptoms of digestive disorders and improve gut health upon consumption.

Supports Liver Detoxification

- **Cleanses the Liver:** The liver is generally the major detoxification organ in the body, filtering out toxins and waste products from the blood. The Castor Oil and Lemon Detox Drink supports liver function by stimulating the production of bile and enhancing the liver's detoxification capability.

- **Reduces Liver Fat:** Lemon juice is alkalizing and thus prevents liver fat, which ensures liver health. The drink helps the liver in its natural detoxification process, enabling it to prevent liver diseases and improve overall health.

Boosts Immunity and Energy Levels

- **Rich in Nutrients:** Lemon juice is rich in vitamin C, among other essential elements required for immunity enhancement and the instillation of vital energy. This drink supports good digestion and detoxification, improving nutrient absorption in the body and leaving you energized and more aggressive.
- **Detoxifies the Body:** Lemon Detox Drink, when consumed together with Castor Oil and on a regular basis, will clean the body from toxins, thereby minimizing the work of the immune system against all other invading toxic forces that are trying to take over and gather inside the body to the degree that diseases manifest.

Aids in Weight Management

Promotes Metabolism: Castor oil and lemon juice work together to increase metabolism, allowing the human body to begin burning fat and keeping weight at a healthy level. The drink also helps eliminate waste, which cuts down on bloating and water retention.

Reduces Appetite: By nature, lemon juice helps suppress appetites; hence, food cravings will be reduced, and one can maintain a healthy diet accordingly. The detox drink will work efficiently for weight-watchers because it helps in digestion and makes them feel fuller.

Improves Skin Health

- **Detoxifies the Skin:** The skin's health is very closely related to detoxification processes in the body, and it is the largest organ that takes part in detoxification. The Castor Oil and Lemon Detox Drink enhances liver function, which helps stimulate the elimination of toxins, thereby improving skin health, reducing acne, and promoting a clear, radiant complexion.
- **Promotes Collagen Production:** Lemon juice is a rich source of vitamin C, which plays an important role in the synthesis of collagen. Collagen keeps skin supple and wrinkle-free. Regular intake of the detox drink delays the onset of premature signs of aging and improves skin texture.

How to Prepare the Castor Oil and Lemon Detox Drink

Ingredients:

- 1 tablespoon of castor oil (cold-pressed and hexane-free)
- Juice of half a fresh lemon (organic if possible)
- 1 cup of warm water
- 1 teaspoon of raw honey or a pinch of cinnamon (optional, for taste)

Instructions:

- **Mix the Ingredients:** In a glass, mix the castor oil, warm water, and freshly squeezed lemon juice. Stir well to combine them properly. To enhance the flavor, add a pinch of cinnamon or a teaspoon of raw honey.

- **Drink on an Empty Stomach:** For maximum efficiency, the castor oil and Lemon Detox Drink must be taken on an empty stomach, preferably early in the morning. This starts the day's detoxification process and allows the nutrients to be better absorbed by the body.
- **Hydrate:** Plenty of water should be drunk throughout the day following the detox drink to help the body's detoxification processes and clear out the toxins.
- **Frequency of Use:** You can take this drink once or twice a week as part of your usual detox program if you are starting to work with castor oil, starting with a little less than that, such as one teaspoonful, gradually increasing your dosage as your body gets used to it.

Precautions and Considerations

Despite the many health advantages of the Castor Oil and Lemon Detox Drink, it's crucial that you use them safely and carefully.

- **Start with a Low Dosage:** If you are new to taking castor oil, it is better to take a reduced dose, one teaspoon, and build up when the body gets used to it. Taking an excess in the initial stages may give rise to discomfort, such as cramps or diarrhea, due to its high laxative effect.
- **Consult with a Healthcare Provider:** If you are planning to undergo a castor oil detox program, consult your health professional in case of pregnancy, lactation, and medication, or if you have

any chronic disorders. It is particularly important for people suffering from liver disorders, gastrointestinal disorders, or intolerance to sharp, acidic food.

- **Hydration is Key:** If castor oil is not taken correctly, its laxative properties can cause dehydration. So remember to drink lots of water during the day when you have this detox drink, keeping yourself hydrated and helping your body flush out the toxins.

- **Avoid Long-Term Use:** The Castor Oil and Lemon Detox Drink is not indicated for long-term use to address any digestive or health issues but is more of a short-term detoxifier. Long-term consumption of castor oil as a laxative may cause habituation and other health adversities. Mix this with other healthy lifestyle habits and consume it once in a while as part of your seasonal detox to help your body naturally eliminate the toxins.

- **Listen to Your Body:** Since everyone reacts to the various detox programs in different ways, it is essential to listen to your own body and adjust your regimen as you see fit. If you experience discomfort or an adverse effect during this time, you must either minimize the dose of the detox drink or the frequency of its application or leave it altogether.

The Castor Oil and Lemon Detox Drink is an all-natural, robust solution for facilitating your body's detoxification processes, enhancing digestion, and improving general well-being. This drink may offer a holistic detoxification method that will help you feel lighter, more energized, and generally healthier. Its alkalizing qualities are derived from lemon juice, and its cleaning qualities are from castor oil.

The Castor Oil and Lemon Detox Drink is an excellent addition to any health program, whether one's objectives are to support the body's natural processes, regulate weight, or stimulate detox. Like any detox program, this drink should be taken with great care and moderation. At the same time, one must continue with a proper intake of nutritious food, regular exercise, and a healthy lifestyle.

In this chapter, we looked at how some of the special qualities of castor oil make it a potent beauty elixir, which can treat everything from stubborn acne to pigmentation. Castor oil offers full and natural skincare, from hydration to anti-aging, acne therapy, and prevention of stretch marks. It is a necessary ingredient in every beauty routine due to the fact that it is versatile, affordable, and effective in its results, without the action of hazardous chemicals. This will continue as the chapter goes on, teaching the reader further on how to use castor oil on the skin, besides ways to balance out healthily, glowing skin naturally.

Chapter 2:
Hair Restoration: Castor Oil to the Rescue for Strong Thick Hair

Castor oil has become an overnight sensation worldwide among hair care lovers for naturally facilitating hair growth, scalp health, and even brow and lash enhancement. It is one such item that should be present in every kit of hair care, considering the high mineral and essential fatty acid content present in it. It also strengthens and revitalizes hair, and specific instructions for the different types of hair and their numerous issues are provided in this chapter.

Castor Oil Application for Hair Growth to Thinning Hair and Hair Loss Reduction

Castor oil has gained a great reputation for its ability to promote hair growth and prevent hair loss. It treats the hair follicles and favors thick hair, giving healthy hair growth; besides being rich in ricinoleic acid, omega-6, and omega-9 fatty acids.

Stimulating Hair Follicles: Smearing castor oil stimulates blood circulation to the scalp, thus activating all idle hair follicles, which eventually produce new hair. Regular massaging of oil into the scalp helps reverse and at least slow down the thinning and falling of hair.

Strengthening Hair Strands: Castor oil acts by strengthening the healthy elements in each hair strand to avoid breakage and split ends. The oil covers brittle or fragile hair like varnish.

Preventing Hair Loss: Castor oil's moisturizing properties keep the strands of hair more flexible and moister, minimizing breakage and the resulting rate of hair loss. The anti-inflammatory properties of castor oil act to soothe scalp disorders like folliculitis, which irritate the scalp and promote hair loss.

Adding castor oil into one's routine can be a very inexpensive and natural remedy for anyone who is experiencing thinning hair or who is losing hair. Use it as a pre-shampoo treatment on the scalp to stimulate hair growth over time, or mix it with other ingredients for a night-time scalp massage.

Homemade Hair Masks: Conditioners and Treatments for All Hair Types

Castor oil, being one of the most versatile oils, provides the perfect base for homemade hair masks designed to target specific hair types and problems. Be it dry, or greasy hair, there's a castor oil remedy that rejuvenates damaged hair.

Dry Hair: Castor oil is thick in viscosity and deeply nourishes dry brittle hair. Use it as a hydrating hair mask with a mix of some coconut or avocado oil. This formula softens hair, replacing lost moisture with shine.

Recipe: Mix 1 tbsp of coconut oil, 2 tbsp of castor oil, and 1 mashed avocado.

Oily Hair: This may go against instincts, but applying oil to oily hair works to balance out oil production in the scalp. Dilute castor oil into lighter oils of jojoba, adding a few drops of tea tree to help clean out the scalp and balance the oil. Recipe: 5 drops of tea tree added to 1 tablespoon of each castor and jojoba

Damaged Hair: Castor oil has restorative properties, which help repair hair that is commonly damaged by chemical treatments, dyeing, or heat styling. It can be used in the making of therapeutic masks with aloe vera and honey for strengthening and treating damaged hair.

Recipe: 2 tablespoons castor oil, 1 tablespoon honey, and 2 tablespoons aloe vera gel.

The advantage of these simple DIY recipes is that they allow everyone to create a hair mask that suits their own needs and serves as a healthier alternative compared to store-bought treatments stuffed with chemicals.

Scalp Care: Dandruff and Scalp Health

Good scalp health is essential for the general health of hair, and castor oil may be fairly effective in treating some of the common scalp conditions, including irritation and dandruff. Castor oil has tremendous, soothing effects on the scalp, due to its antifungal and antibacterial nature, and it creates very suitable conditions for hair growth.

Treating Dandruff: Generally, the principal cause of dandruff may be a dry scalp; thus, it may be prevented by using the moisturizing properties of castor oil. Antifungal properties of castor oil prevent fungal infections, which are responsible for dandruff while soothing irritation and flaking of the scalp after being applied topically.

Procedure: Massage scalp with castor oil, adding a few drops of tea tree oil. Leave it on for half an hour before shampooing to help soften dandruff on the scalp and reduce it.

Increasing Blood Flow to the Scalp: Castor oil applied to the scalp increases blood flow, which is necessary to stimulate hair growth. It moisturizes the skin as well. Increased blood flow ensures that the nutrients required by hair follicles to produce healthy and strong hair get delivered.

Anti-Inflammation Benefits: Anti-inflammatory properties of the castor oil soothe itching, redness, and inflammation associated with psoriasis and eczema over the scalp. So, it is ideal for tender scalp care.

Frequent masses of castor oil on the scalp will keep it healthy and maintain a proper balance of the scalp, reducing problems like dandruff and will provide a very suitable environment for hair growth.

Scalp Treatment for Hair Growth

Hair growth starts at a healthy scalp. A healthy and nourished scalp keeps a perfect balance to help the hair follicles grow properly, thus stimulating thick, complete, and shiny hair. Stress, poor nutrition, and changes in hormones are detriments to scalp health, while using inappropriate hair products ultimately creates thinning hair, slow growth, and hair loss. Fortunately, natural remedies like castor oil are blended with specific essential oils and herbal infusions to resolve these issues. This chapter discusses three highly effective scalp treatments for stimulating hair growth using castor oil: Peppermint & Castor Oil Hair Growth Booster, Herbal Infusion Castor Oil Scalp Massage, and Cinnamon Castor Scalp Stimulant.

Peppermint & Castor Oil Hair Growth Booster
Why It Works

Peppermint oil is renowned for its therapeutic and stimulating effects. It is used topically on the scalp to enhance flow, thereby ensuring your hair follicles get the much-needed oxygen and nutrients for growth. Secondly, it has a soothing, cooling effect that reduces scalp irritation and inflammation—two of the major culprits in hair loss. A blend with castor oil, which deeply nourishes and strengthens hair, will be an excellent combination to enhance hair growth and scalp health.

Benefits

- **Stimulates Hair Growth:** Peppermint oil is composed of menthol, which acts as a vasodilator. It widens the blood vessels to enable more blood flow to the scalp. This, in turn, allows such increased circulation to supply all the nutrients to the hair follicles, stimulating their growth.
- **Strengthens Hair:** Castor oil is rich in fatty acids, with a high concentration of ricinoleic acid, that strengthen hair from the root, reduce hair breakage, and improve elasticity.
- **Soothes and Conditions the Scalp:** Peppermint oil's anti-inflammatory properties reduce irritation or itchiness on the scalp, while castor oil conditions and nourish the scalp to avoid dryness and flakiness.

How to Make and Use the Peppermint & Castor Oil Hair Growth Booster

Ingredients:

- 2 tablespoons of castor oil (cold-pressed and hexane-free)
- 5-7 drops of peppermint essential oil
- 1 tablespoon of coconut oil (optional, for added moisture)
- A small, clean bottle or jar for storage

Instructions:

- **Combine the Oils:** In a small bowl, mix the castor oil with the peppermint essential oil. If you have very dry or fragile hair, you may add a tablespoon of coconut oil to the mixture to add extra hydration.
- **Transfer to a Bottle:** Pour into a small clean bottle or jar with a tight-fitting lid. At this point, shake the bottle well to combine the oils.
- **Application:** Apply the treatment to dry scalp and hair. Section your hair to apply it more evenly. Lightly massage the oil mixture into your scalp with your fingertips, paying particular attention to areas of thinning or slow growth. Massage for 5 to 10 minutes to stimulate blood flow.
- **Leave On:** To get the maximum benefit, leave the treatment on your scalp for at least 30 minutes. You can also keep it overnight by wrapping your hair in a shower cap to save your bedding.
- **Rinse and Shampoo:** After keeping it on for the prescribed time, wash your hair thoroughly with warm water, followed by shampooing to remove the oil.

Usage Tips:

- This may be done once or twice a week to stimulate hair growth and calm the scalp.
- If your skin is sensitive, you can use a lower dilution of peppermint essential oil to avoid irritation.

Herbal Infusion Castor Oil Scalp Massage
Why It Works

Herbal infusions are an ancient technique for extracting valuable properties from plants for hair care. The addition of these herbs, which are known to infuse castor oil with hair-enhancing and hair-growth properties, makes this concoction an effective treatment for the scalp. It strengthens the roots of hair and is soon followed by healthy hair growth. Indeed, this treatment features castor oil at the forefront, along with other herbs like rosemary, lavender, and nettle that are well-known for their benefits for hair and scalp health.

Benefits

- **Deep Nourishment:** Herbal infusion profoundly nourishes the scalp with a concentrated dose of vitamins, minerals, and antioxidants for deep nourishment and strengthening hair follicles.
- **Stimulates Hair Growth:** Herbs such as rosemary and nettle stimulate hair growth by improving circulation and feeding hair follicles with all the essential nutrients.
- **Reduces Hair Loss:** Lavender's active ingredient combines with other calming herbs to balance scalp

oil production and soothe irritation, reducing hair loss caused by stress or inflammation.

How to Make and Use the Herbal Infusion Castor Oil Scalp Massage

Ingredients:

- 1/2 cup of castor oil (cold-pressed and hexane-free)
- 1 tablespoon of dried rosemary
- 1 tablespoon of dried lavender
- 1 tablespoon of dried nettle
- A glass jar with a lid for infusion
- A small, clean bottle for storage

Instructions:

- **Create the Herbal Infusion:** Prepare the glass jar by adding the herbs, rosemary, lavender, and nettle. Then, pour the castor oil into the jar to cover the herbs.
- **Infuse the Oil:** Place the jar in a warm, sunny spot with the lid sealed. Shake the jar gently every few days to allow for the infusion process. The longer the herbs are allowed to infuse into the oil, the more potent it will be.
- **Strain the Oil:** In 2 weeks, strain the oil through a fine mesh sieve or cheesecloth into a clean bottle, discarding the herbs. Your herbal-infused castor oil is ready for application.
- **Application:** Apply this infused oil by warming up a small amount in your hands and massaging it into the scalp. Using your fingertips, massage the scalp with a circular motion, paying special attention to

those areas where hair growth is desired or where the scalp is dry or irritated.

- **Leave On:** Apply the oil to your scalp and leave it on for at least 30 minutes or overnight for an intense treatment. To prevent your bedding from staining, cover your hair with a shower cap or even a towel for the night.
- **Rinse and Shampoo:** After the treatment, rinse well using lukewarm water and shampoo your hair to eliminate the oil residue.

Usage Tips:

- The treatment is beneficial if taken once a week in order to nourish the scalp and give good nourishment to the hair for healthy growth.
- Store the infused oil in a cool, dark place to preserve its potency.

Cinnamon Castor Scalp Stimulant
Why It Works

When applied topically, this highly active spice stimulates and increases the flow of blood. Increased blood flow means the hair follicles get more nutrients and oxygen, hence the faster growth rate. When combined with castor oil, which deeply moisturizes and nourishes hair, cinnamon creates a warming, invigorating scalp treatment that can jumpstart growth and revitalize tired, thinning hair.

Benefits

- **Stimulates Blood Flow:** Cinnamon stimulates blood flow to the scalp, activating hair follicles and encouraging hair growth.
- **Strengthens Hair Follicles:** The combination of cinnamon and castor oil helps strengthen hair follicles. As a result, there will be less breakage and shedding, which means more hair will remain on the head.
- **Balances Scalp Oils:** Cinnamon also possesses antimicrobial properties that help balance scalp oils, preventing conditions such as dandruff or any scalp conditions that inhibit hair growth.

How to Make and Use the Cinnamon Castor Scalp Stimulant

Ingredients:

- 2 tablespoons of castor oil (cold-pressed and hexane-free)
- 1 teaspoon of ground cinnamon or 3-5 drops of cinnamon essential oil
- 1 tablespoon of olive oil or almond oil (optional, for added moisture)
- A small, clean bottle or jar for storage

Instructions:

- **Combine the Ingredients:** In a small bowl, mix castor oil with ground cinnamon or cinnamon essential oil. If you want a lighter treatment, dilute the mixture further with olive or almond oil.
- **Transfer to a Bottle:** Pour the mixture into a small, clean bottle or jar and shake well to combine.

- **Application:** Apply this to a clean, dry scalp. Segment your hair and apply the mixture directly to your scalp with your fingertips. Massage the oil into your scalp in circular motions at areas where you want to stimulate growth.
- **Leave On:** Leave the treatment on for 20 to 30 minutes. You might feel the warming of the cinnamon; this is quite normal, as it stimulates the blood flow.
- **Rinse and Shampoo:** Rinse your hair liberally with lukewarm water. Then, use your regular shampoo and conditioner to remove the oil.

Usage Tips:

- This treat could be applied once every week to keep your scalp in good condition and stimulate hair growth.
- If you experience any irritation or discomfort, reduce the amount of cinnamon in the mixture or shorten the application time.

Wholesome, thick, and radiant hair growth starts from scalp care. These three scalp treatments-namely Peppermint & Castor Oil Hair Growth Booster, Herbal Infusion Castor Oil Scalp Massage, and Cinnamon Castor Scalp Stimulant-nourish the scalp, stimulate hair follicles, and promote robust hair growth. Each of these treatments capitalizes on the natural efficiency of castor oil in concert with other potent ingredients to handle specific scalp and hair needs.

Incorporated into regular hair care, these treatments encourage significant improvements in hair growth and texture and help keep the scalp in good health. Whether one faces hair thinning, poor scalp health, or even aspires for more robust hair growth, these natural remedies effectively solve such problems without using chemicals. Keep using them, and in no time, you will be on the right path towards healthy and fantastic hair, which you have always wished for.

Dandruff Remedy Shampoo

Dandruff is a scalp disorder that appears as an uncontrollable shedding of the outermost layer of the scalp in noticeable amounts, often accompanied by itching and irritation. It has been attributed to an oily or dry scalp, fungal infections, and even an allergic reaction to hair care products. While dandruff is rarely, if ever, a health concern, it is often uncomfortable and embarrassing. Most commercial anti-dandruff shampoos have harsh chemicals that may further irritate the scalp or strip the hair of its natural oils. Castor oil and other potent ingredients will help soothe the scalp and reduce flaking to develop a healthy scalp environment. This section looks into four of the best dandruff remedy shampoos that incorporate castor oil: Lemon Zest Castor Oil Dandruff Fighter, Apple Cider & Castor Soothing Shampoo, Neem & Castor Scalp Purifying Shampoo, and Charcoal & Castor Deep-Cleansing Shampoo.

Lemon Zest Castor Oil Dandruff Fighter
Why It Works

Lemon zest is rich in citric acid, an antifungal and antibacterial agent that naturally fights against the common yeast and bacteria that accompany dandruff. The astringent action of lemon helps reduce excess oil on the scalp, which contributes to the problem. In combination with castor oil's moisturizing and anti-inflammatory properties, this shampoo will clean the scalp to reduce flakiness while leaving hair fresh and invigorated.

Benefits

- **Reduces Flaking:** Lemon's citric acid exfoliates your scalp by loosening dead skin cells, thus reducing flaking.
- **Balances Scalp Oil:** Lemon's astringent properties help regulate the scalp's oil production, preventing oil build-up and dandruff.
- **Moisturizes and Soothes:** Castor oil hydrates with moisturizing effectiveness, soothing irritation and inflammation sometimes associated with dandruff.

How to Make and Use the Lemon Zest Castor Oil Dandruff Fighter

Ingredients:

- 2 tablespoons of castor oil (cold-pressed and hexane-free)
- Zest of 1 lemon
- Juice of half a lemon
- 1/4 cup of liquid castile soap (unscented)
- 10 drops of tea tree essential oil (optional, for additional antifungal properties)
- A clean bottle for storage

Instructions:

- **Prepare the Lemon Zest:** Grate the lemon using a fine grater; be careful not to grate any white pith because it is pretty bitter. Squeeze half of the lemon for its juice.

- **Mix the Ingredients:** In one bowl, mix the castor oil, lemon zest, lemon juice, and liquid castile soap. If preferred, add the tea tree essential oil. Mix well so that the ingredients combine properly.
- **Transfer to a Bottle:** Transfer the mixture into a clean, tight-lidded bottle. Shake well before every use to combine the ingredients.
- **Application:** Shampoo on wet hair mainly focuses on the scalp. Gently massage for 2 to 3 minutes to let the magic of lemon and castor oil act on the scalp. Rinse well using lukewarm water.
- **Condition and Rinse:** Follow with your usual conditioner or an apple cider vinegar rinse to further balance the scalp pH and add shine to your hair.

Usage Tips:

- This shampoo should be used two to three times a week to combat dandruff and maintain your scalp in its best condition.
- For more prolonged use, keep the shampoo in a cool, dark place.

Apple Cider & Castor Soothing Shampoo
Why It Works

Apple cider vinegar, commonly called ACV, is among those naturals famous for balancing scalp pH and impeding the growth of fungi and bacteria. Its acidity exfoliates the scalp and removes the dead skin cells, which reduces the flakes brought on by dandruff. Added to castor oil, which provides dry nourishment with anti-inflammatory benefits, this shampoo calms the scalp and is naturally perfect for hair to grow. Benefits.

Benefits

- Balances Scalp pH: Apple cider vinegar helps restore the scalp's natural pH balance, which, if not too acidic or too alkaline, can help avoid dandruff.
- Fights Fungal Infections: ACV's antifungal property fights the yeast and fungi that could cause flaking due to dandruff, which minimizes itchiness and flakiness.
- Moisturizes and Conditions: Castor oil deeply moisturizes the scalp, avoiding dryness and further flaking while soothing irritation.

How to Make and Use the Apple Cider & Castor Soothing Shampoo

Ingredients:

- 2 tablespoons of castor oil (cold-pressed and hexane-free)
- 1/4 cup of apple cider vinegar (organic, with the "mother")
- 1/4 cup of distilled water
- 1/4 cup of liquid castile soap (unscented)
- 5 drops of rosemary essential oil (optional, for additional scalp health benefits)
- A clean bottle for storage

Instructions:

- **Mix the Ingredients:** Castor oil, apple cider vinegar, distilled water, and liquid castile soap in a bowl.

Rosemary essential oil can be added if desired. Stir well to ensure that it is well mixed.

- **Transfer to a Bottle:** Pour the mixture into a clean bottle with a tight-fitting lid. Always shake the bottle before use to mix the ingredients.
- **Application:** Apply the shampoo on wet hair directly on the scalp. Gently massage in a circular motion for 2-3 minutes to allow the ACV and castor oil to penetrate the scalp. Rinse with thoroughly lukewarm water.
- **Condition and Rinse:** Follow with a conditioner to lock in moisture. You can also use an ACV rinse diluted 1 part ACV to 4 parts water as a final rinse to add shine and further balance the scalp's pH.

Usage Tips:

- Use this shampoo 2-3 times a week to maintain a dandruff-free scalp and promote healthy hair growth.
- Store the shampoo in a cool, dark place to preserve its effectiveness.

Neem & Castor Scalp Purifying Shampoo
Why It Works

Neem oil is a potent extract derived from neem tree seeds. It offers antifungal, antibacterial, and anti-inflammatory properties. In Ayurvedic medicine, neem has been used for hundreds of years to treat various scalp and skin disorders, such as dandruff. Blended with castor oil, neem oil cleans the scalp of impurities, lessening flakiness and irritation. Therefore, it would be an excellent mixture to cure chronic dandruff.

Benefits

- **Purifies the Scalp:** It cleanses the scalp, clearing all impurities and reducing fungus and bacteria that could lead to dandruff.
- **Reduces Inflammation:** The anti-inflammatory properties of neem soothe the scalp by reducing redness, itchiness, and irritation from dandruff.
- **Strengthens Hair Follicles:** Neem, mixed with castor oil, helps strengthen hair follicles, which inhibits hair loss and offers healthy hair growth.

How to Make and Use the Neem & Castor Scalp Purifying Shampoo

Ingredients:

- 2 tablespoons of castor oil (cold-pressed and hexane-free)
- 1 tablespoon of neem oil (organic, cold-pressed)
- 1/4 cup of liquid castile soap (unscented)
- 1/4 cup of distilled water
- 5 drops of peppermint essential oil (optional, for a refreshing scent and additional scalp stimulation)
- A clean bottle for storage

Instructions:

- Mix the Ingredients: In a bowl, mix together castor oil, neem oil, liquid castile soap, and distilled water. Peppermint essential oil can be added if desired. Stir the mixture until all contents are well incorporated.
- Transfer to a Bottle: Pour this into a clean bottle with a tight-fitting lid. Always shake before each use to combine the ingredients.

- Application: Apply the shampoo to wet hair, massaging mostly the scalp. Massage lightly for 2-3 minutes to allow neem oil and castor oil to clean and purify the scalp. Rinse with plenty of lukewarm water.
- Condition and Rinse: Then apply your regular conditioner or a neem-based conditioner that will give an added touch to the purification action. Rinse with cool water to seal the hair cuticle and add shine.

Usage Tips:

- Use this shampoo 1-2 times a week for a deep scalp cleanse and to keep dandruff at bay.
- Store the shampoo in a cool, dark place to maintain its potency.

Charcoal & Castor Deep-Cleansing Shampoo
Why It Works

Activated charcoal is a powerful detoxifying agent that may be able to draw out impurities, toxins, and excess oil from the scalp. This will be especially effective for people with oily scalps or those who use a lot of hair products, as it deeply cleanses the scalp and avoids any buildup that may lead to dandruff. Blended with castor oil, this deep-cleansing shampoo helps to moisturize and soothe the scalp, evening out the approach in an effort to fight dandruff and ensure a healthy scalp environment.

Benefits

- **Detoxifies the Scalp:** Activated charcoal acts like a magnet, drawing out dirt, oil, and impurities from the scalp, leaving it fresh and clean.
- **Reduces Buildup:** A shampoo is great at removing buildup from various hair products that might clog hair follicles and cause dandruff or other scalp problems.
- **Moisturizes and Nourishes:** Castor oil gives the scalp the much-needed moisture, preventing it from drying out and flaking off. It also comforts irritated areas.

How to Make and Use the Charcoal & Castor Deep-Cleansing Shampoo

Ingredients:

- 2 tablespoons of castor oil (cold-pressed and hexane-free)
- 1 tablespoon of activated charcoal powder
- 1/4 cup of liquid castile soap (unscented)
- 1/4 cup of distilled water
- 5 drops of tea tree essential oil (optional, for its antifungal properties)
- A clean bottle for storage

Instructions:

- **Mix the Ingredients:** In a bowl, mix the castor oil, activated charcoal powder, liquid castile soap, and distilled water. If using, add the tea tree essential oil. Ensure all the ingredients are well combined.

- **Transfer to a Bottle:** Pour the mixture into a clean, dark-tinted bottle with a tight-fitting lid. Always shake before use to combine ingredients.
- **Application:** Apply the shampoo to the wet hair, scalp-oriented. Massage gently for 2-3 minutes, allowing the activated charcoal and castor oil to clean and detoxify the scalp. Afterward, rinse your hair with lukewarm water.
- **Condition and Rinse:** To restore moisture and smoothness, nourish the hair with a conditioner. Then, rinse it with cold water to close the cuticles and lock moisture in.

Usage Tips:

- Use this shampoo once a week for a deep cleanse, especially if you have an oily scalp or use a lot of styling products.
- Store the shampoo in a cool, dark place to preserve its effectiveness.

Dandruff is a chronic and frustrating problem; it can be controlled, even eradicated, with perfect natural remedies. In a nutshell, the following dandruff treatment shampoos- Lemon Zest Castor Oil Dandruff Fighter, Apple Cider & Castor Soothing Shampoo, Neem & Castor Scalp Purifying Shampoo, and Charcoal & Castor Deep Cleansing Shampoo-offer potent natural options to salons full of chemical-laden commercial products. Each shampoo is designed to combat the roots of the causes leading to dandruff-from excess oil, product buildup, and fungal infection to imbalanced scalp pH.

These shampoos will help significantly improve scalp health, reduce flaking, and create more robust and healthier hair. Treatment with natural ingredients such as castor oil, lemon zest, apple cider vinegar, neem, and activated charcoal is all one needs to get a healthy and balanced scalp and enjoy dandruff-free hair. Whether one needs an everyday gentle shampoo or a treatment for deep cleansing, these recipes are the way to go in maintaining a healthy, no-flake scalp.

How to Get Longer Eyelashes and Fuller Brows and Lash Growth

Castor oil is now seen as a solution for people who want longer eyelashes and fuller eyebrows, aside from hair and scalp care. The nutrients in castor oil help with the hair growth of such definite areas and are healthy alternatives to harsh chemicals or treatments.

Fuller Brows: Castor oil is great for reviving sparse eyebrows, which could be due to excessive plucking or natural balding of hair. With time, you might develop fuller and thicker eyebrows by stimulating hair growth with frequent application of the oil to the brows.

Application Method: Apply castor oil to the eyebrows every night using a clean cotton swab or mascara wand. Results usually appear after a few weeks of constant use.

Longer, Thicker Lashes: To stimulate the length and thickness, castor oil is also able to be used for lashes. The same moisturizing properties that stimulate scalp hair growth work well for delicate lash hairs.

Application Method: Apply a small amount of castor oil to your eyelashes with a clean mascara wand or brush before bedtime. Be careful to avoid getting any oil in your eyes.

Continuously, castor oil is a less expensive, natural alternative for anyone looking to take their lash and eyebrow game to the next level without the added expenses of serums or extensions.

This chapter has discussed various benefits concerning castor oil for hair health, including how it can improve brows and lashes, treat scalp conditions, and even stimulate hair growth while slowing down hair loss. Castor oil is a miracle worker to make hair healthy, and thick, and solve the common problems related to hair due to its natural extracts and nutritional values. Castor oil is thus flexible and effective for every hair type, whether applied alone or as a part of homemade hair treatments. As readers progress through this book, they will be enlightened with new uses of this miraculous oil in making over general health and appearance.

Chapter 3:
DIY Castor Oil Recipes for Beautifying Yourself

Castor Oil Skincare is really trending toward more green and natural alternatives in the beauty industry. Because castor oil has moisturizing and anti-inflammatory benefits and also blends rather easily with other natural elements, it can serve as the base to create personalized beauty products. This chapter provides the reader with some useful and easy-to-make recipes, which avail benefits of castor oil in creating natural beauty products for hand lotions, lip balms, moisturizers, and many others. In addition to the safety precautions given to ensure consumption safety, we shall also take a look at the safe admixture of castor oil with other carrier oils and essential oils.

Natural Cleansers, Moisturizers, and Serums

Castor oil is known to be so good at locking moisture in that it makes a great base for homemade skin care products. Castor oil deeply nourishes the skin not only by preserving the barrier of the skin by preserving its moisture but also due to the high content of fatty acids and vitamin E that it possesses. The following section will guide the readers through preparing natural moisturizers, cleansers, and serums with castor oil as their main ingredient.

DIY Your Moisturizer: Castor oil blended with other nourishing moisturizing ingredients like aloe vera or jojoba oil creates an intensely nourishing, non-comedogenic moisturizer. The perfect formulation for sensitive, acne-prone skin types, it is ideal for day-long moisturization without clogged pores.

Recipe: Mix 1 tablespoon of aloe vera gel with 2 tablespoons of castor oil and 1 tablespoon of jojoba oil. Stir well and apply for a regular face cream.

Skin Cleanser: Using oil on the skin is one of the favored methods for maintaining healthy and hydrated skin. Castor oil is very suitable as a cleanser, as it does not strip the skin of its natural oils because of the simple fact that it will just break down extra oil and impurities.

Recipe: Mix 1 tablespoon of olive oil with 2 tablespoons of castor oil. Massage over dry skin for a few minutes, then remove using a warm towel.

Anti-Aging Serum: The richness of antioxidants in castor oil helps to fight free radicals and prevent early aging. This, therefore, makes it perfect for use in a very potent anti-aging serum, combined with such essential oils as rosehip or frankincense, which plump up fine wrinkles and encourage younger-looking skin.

Recipe: Take a tablespoon of castor oil, add to it a tablespoon of rosehip oil, and 5 drops of essential frankincense oil. Apply every night to see visible results.

These homemade skincare creams provide you with a customized skincare formula according to your skin needs help you completely control what you put onto your skin and avoid harmful chemicals often found in over-the-counter products.

Making Your Hand Creams and Lip Balms

Castor oil is an ideal ingredient for lip balms and hand creams, as its viscosity is thick, making it perfect to be applied in order to create a barrier on the skin. It is an active component in this cosmetic because it helps deeply hydrate and comfort dry hands and chapped lips.

Lip Balm: Commercial lip balms are loaded with artificial ingredients that often just give symptom relief without hydration or repair of the lips. This homemade lip balm with castor oil prevents drying of the lips by keeping them hydrated continuously, especially during bad weather.

Castor oil 1 tbsp, Beeswax 1 tbsp, Shea butter 1 tbsp, Essential peppermint oil 5 drops. To make cooling lip balm, the beeswax, and shea butter are melted in a pan kept at low heat, and the castor oil with the melted product, adding essential oil to it.

Hand Cream: Castor oil is good for making homemade hand cream, particularly for dry, cracked hands, due to the oil's ability to lock in moisture in one's hands. This can be mixed with other emollients like coconut oil and shea butter to create a nourishing, soothing, and protective hand cream.

Castor oil - 2 tablespoons, shea butter - 2 tablespoons, and coconut oil - 1 tablespoon. Mix the shea butter with coconut oil in advance; then add castor oil and let it cool.

Besides saving money, one thing is for sure: hand creams and lip balms will be free from dangerous additives, being pure and effective hydration and protection for one's skin.

Castor Oil Blended with Other Carrier Oils for Maximum Efficiency

While castor oil is very potent on its own, it may be used in combination with other oils to further extend the efficacy of castor oil for certain skin and scalp disorders. The following section examines how different carrier oil combinations can be applied for the purpose of targeting specific skin issues relating to aging, inflammation, and dryness.

Castor Oil + Jojoba Oil: This oil combination may help in regulating the amount of sebum your skin produces and keep your oily or acne-prone skin hydrated but light. Jojoba oil is the best for oily skin because it comes closest to your skin's natural oils.

Benefit: Not only does it keep acne away, but it also keeps your skin moisturized without leaving your skin greasy.

Usage: This night facial oil can be used with a castor and jojoba oil mixture in a 1:1 ratio.

Castor Oil + Argan Oil: The combination is an effective hydrating and antioxidant action on dry or aged skin. Argan oil has a high vitamin E content, which enhances the hydrating properties of castor oil; hence, it is suitable for dry or aged skin.

Benefits: Reduces wrinkles, makes the skin supple, and deeply nourishes it.

Use a mixture of castor and argan oil in a 1:2 ratio as a moisturizer or sleeping mask overnight.

Castor oil with sweet almond oil is very calming because of the presence of ingredients that calm irritation, thus lightening the skin without leaving it greasy. Almond oil has healthy skin-promoting vitamins and minerals, such as vitamins A and E, to keep your skin healthy without any sensitivity or breakout.

Benefits: Soothing effect on redness and irritation, maintains hydration of the skin.

How to use it: Mix 1 part castor oil with 2 parts almond oil and use it as a daily face oil for sensitive skin.

By balancing castor oil with different base oils, readers can increase the benefits for their individual skin and hair problems and develop a personalized skincare routine for themselves.

Safety and Side Effects: A Word of Caution

While castor oil has a number of beautifying benefits, proper administration will help one avoid its numerous adverse implications. Even though it is generally regarded harmless, improper application or its excess may bring about some kind of adverse effects. Safety precautions, probable adverse effects, and recommended usage of castor oil are discussed here.

This is an important step, before the application of castor oil or its derivatives to the skin surface in large numbers. It is done by applying a little of it on the inner arm or wrist and waiting 24 hours for observation of any allergic reaction. Common Reactions: Typically, itching, erythema, or irritation is quite unusual but could occur in some sensitive individuals. If it does, one simply should not use it.

Dilution for Sensitive Skin: Castor oil can be quite thick and may be too heavy at times for sensitive skin types. One can dilute it with lighter oils such as coconut or jojoba oil, making the solution more acceptable for normal use, without being overpowering to the skin.

It is recommended that one dilutes castor oil 1:2 with a milder carrier oil in cases of sensitive skin.

For Internal Use Caution: Castor oil, though claimed many times to be a remedy for constipation, should only be used under a doctor's consultation because an overdose of this may lead to severe cramps, diarrhea, or dehydration.

Eye Contact: While applying castor oil on eyebrows or eyelashes, beware lest it enters into the eyes. Wash your eyes properly in case this happens. This might result in irritation/discomfort caused by the prolonged touch of castor oil on the delicate parts of your body.

Eczema and Psoriasis Soothing Blends

Eczema and psoriasis are chronic skin diseases, often accompanied by significant discomfort, irritation, and distress. Each of these diseases involves inflammation, skin redness, itching feelings, and flaking. Though there is no cure for eczema or psoriasis, natural home remedies can soothe symptoms and reduce inflammation by encouraging the healing process. Castor oil is one of the most potent ingredients in the treatment of such diseases due to its anti-inflammatory, moisturizing, and healing properties. Castor oil can be combined with other natural mainstays to make a few effective soothing blends that would alleviate symptoms of eczema and psoriasis. This section looks at five blends that will help harness the power of castor oil to meet the other skin-loving ingredients.

Oatmeal & Castor Oil Eczema Relief Paste
Why It Works:

Oatmeal is famous for its anti-inflammatory and soothing properties, which is why it's commonly applied to skin issues like eczema. It helps to reduce itching, subside the redness, and moisturize the dry and irritated skin. Castor oil completes the action of oatmeal by moisturizing the skin from deep inside and building a protective barrier, locking moisture inside. In such a way, this combination not only soothes the skin but heals it, too, and avoids further irritation.

Ingredients:

- 2 tablespoons of finely ground oatmeal (colloidal oatmeal is ideal)
- 1 tablespoon of castor oil (cold-pressed and hexane-free)
- 1 teaspoon of honey (optional, for added moisture)
- Warm water (enough to form a paste)

Instructions:

- **Prepare the Oatmeal:** If you are using regular oatmeal, then take it in a blender or food processor and blend to a fine consistency. You may also use colloidal oatmeal, which is pre-ground and ready to use.
- **Mix the Ingredients:** In a small bowl, mix the ground oatmeal and castor oil. Then, add small amounts of warm water, only that much, to form a thick paste. If desired, mix in the honey to enhance the moisturizing effect.

- **Application:** Apply the paste on the affected areas of your skin, massaging it light enough to go even. Leave on the skin for 15-20 minutes.
- **Rinse and Moisturize:** Rinse off the paste with lukewarm water, then pat dry your skin lightly. Follow up with a gentle moisturizer or a thin layer of castor oil that seals in moisture.

Usage Tips:

- Use this paste 2-3 times a week to help soothe eczema flare-ups and maintain healthy, hydrated skin.
- Store any leftover paste in an airtight container in the refrigerator for up to a week. Reheat gently before use.

Castor Oil & Shea Butter Psoriasis Salve
Why It Works:

Psoriasis is a chronic autoimmune disease with rapid skin cell growth symptoms, causing thick, scaly patches that can feel itchy and painful. Shea butter is richly intensive with ingredients that deeply moisturize and soften skin. Blended together with castor oil, whose anti-inflammatory properties are highly attuned to stimulating the healing process, this salve is just what the disease sufferer needs.

Ingredients:

- 2 tablespoons of castor oil (cold-pressed and hexane-free)
- 2 tablespoons of shea butter (raw and unrefined)

- 1 tablespoon of coconut oil (optional, for added moisture)
- 5 drops of lavender essential oil (optional, for calming effects)
- 3 drops of tea tree essential oil (optional, for its antifungal properties)

Instructions:

- Melt the Shea Butter: In a double boiler, melt the shea butter until it reaches a fluid consistency. If using, add coconut oil at this stage to melt along with shea butter.
- Mix in Castor Oil: Remove from heat and stir in the castor oil until well combined.
- Add Essential Oils: If using, add the lavender and tea tree essential oils and mix well.
- Cooling and Solidifying: Pour the mixture into a small, clean container and let it cool to solidify at room temperature or in the refrigerator.
- Application: Apply this salve on the areas with psoriasis as desired, rubbing it into the skin using a gentle massage.

Usage Tips:

- Use the salve daily to keep psoriasis patches moisturized, reduce scaling, and relieve itching.
- Store the salve in a cool, dry place. It can last up to six months if kept in an airtight container.

Calendula & Castor Oil Itch-Relief Balm
Why It Works:

Calendula, commonly known as pot marigold, is a medicating plant that has been used for ages to soothe skin. It is especially effective in reducing inflammation and promoting wound healing. When combined with castor oil, calendula can create a potent balm that soothes itching associated not only with eczema and psoriasis but also with the restoration and cure of damaged skin.

Ingredients:

- 1/4 cup of castor oil (cold-pressed and hexane-free)
- 1/4 cup of calendula-infused oil (you can make this by infusing dried calendula flowers in a carrier oil like olive oil)
- 1 tablespoon of beeswax pellets (for consistency)
- 5 drops of chamomile essential oil (optional, for additional soothing)

Instructions:

- Melt the Beeswax: In a double boiler, heat the beeswax pellets over low heat until melted.
- Add Oils: Add castor oil and calendula-infused oil to the melted beeswax and mix until well incorporated.
- Add Essential Oils: Let cool, remove from heat, and add the chamomile essential oil, if desired.
- Pour and Cool: Pour the mixture into a small, clean jar or clean tin. Let cool and solidify.
- Application: Apply the balm to itchy or inflamed areas when needed. Gently rub it in to soothe and promote healing immediately.

Usage Tips:

- Apply this balm as often as needed, especially during flare-ups to reduce itching and irritation.
- Store the balm in a cool, dark place. It should last for several months if kept in an airtight container.

Cucumber & Castor Oil Skin Calming Cream
Why It Works:

Cucumber is a natural astringent that cools down. Its anti-inflammatory properties are best for soothing irritated skin. It works wonderfully in diminishing redness and calming inflamed skin, including skin from eczema and psoriasis. Moreover, when blended with castor oil, which deeply moisturizes and heals skin, it can treat sensitive skin with the coolest and most soothing treatment.

Ingredients:

- 1/4 cup of castor oil (cold-pressed and hexane-free)
- 1/2 cucumber, peeled and pureed
- 1 tablespoon of aloe vera gel (optional, for added hydration)
- 5 drops of peppermint essential oil (optional, for cooling effect)

Instructions:

- **Prepare the Cucumber:** Peel and puree half a cucumber in a blender or food processor. Line the blender or a bowl with cheesecloth or a thin, clean cotton cloth, and strain out as much liquid from the puree as possible to obtain a thick cucumber pulp.

- **Mix Ingredients:** Mix cucumber pulp, castor oil, and aloe vera gel together in a small bowl. Stir well to combine. Add peppermint essential oil, if desired.
- **Application:** Apply the cream to the affected area and gently massage it into the skin. Leave the cream on for 15-20 minutes, then wash off with cool water.
- **Storage:** Place any remaining cream in an airtight container and store it in the refrigerator. Use within one week.

Usage Tips:

- Use this cream 2-3 times a week, or as needed, to calm irritated skin and reduce redness.
- The cooling effect of cucumber and peppermint makes this cream particularly soothing for flare-ups during warmer weather.

Chamomile Castor Soothe Formula
Why It Works:

Chamomile is known for its antiphlogistic, antiseptic, anti-infective, and sedative effects; thus, it is used to treat excited skin conditions, including eczema and psoriasis. In combination, castor oil with chamomile increases the soothing effects on irritated skin and accelerates healing by offering quick relief from itching, redness, and inflammation.

Ingredients:

- 1/4 cup of castor oil (cold-pressed and hexane-free)

- 1/4 cup of chamomile-infused oil (you can make this by infusing dried chamomile flowers in a carrier oil like olive oil)
- 1 tablespoon of coconut oil (optional, for added moisture)
- 10 drops of chamomile essential oil (for an extra soothing effect)

Instructions:

- **Melt the Coconut Oil:** If using, gently warm the coconut oil in a double boiler.
- **Mix Oils:** Add the castor oil and the chamomile steeped oil to the melted coconut oil if using stirring well.
- **Add Essential Oil:** Remove from heat and add the chamomile essential oil.
- **Application:** Use on affected areas, rubbing into the skin gently to ensure deep absorption. Allow the formula to stay on the skin or rinse off after a few hours.
- **Storage:** Now, let the formula cool down and store it in a dark place. If kept in an airtight container, it will last up to six months.

Usage Tips:

- Apply this formula daily or as needed to soothe and calm irritated skin, reduce inflammation, and relieve itching.
- This formula can also be used as an overnight treatment, leaving it on the skin to work its magic while you sleep.

Eczema and psoriasis are both conditions that are not easy to handle; therefore, with the proper natural remedies, symptoms will be soothed, and further improvement in the health of your skin will be achieved. Recipes in this section merge castor oil's therapeutic properties with other effective natural ingredients to relieve the itching, redness, and inflammation associated with these chronic skin conditions. Each of these comforting blends goes a long way in keeping your skin healthier, calmer, and more robust. The main difference in any treatment is consistency. This will yield optimal results in frequent application, enabling one to avoid flare-ups and maintain comfortable, hydrated skin.

Castor Oil and Banana Hair Conditioner: A Deeply Nourishing Treatment for Luscious Locks

Although a head full of healthy, lively hair is considered by many to be a beauty asset and a sign of life, it is genuinely not easy to acquire and maintain with all the damages brought about by the environment, heat styling, and chemical treatments. The conditioner will nourish against dryness, frizz, and breakage, using such organic ingredients as castor oil and banana. This effectively feeds the hair, strengthens it, and provides a natural shine and softness that often evades commercially prepared products. We shall next consider the benefits of using castor oil and bananas as hair conditioners and describe how to prepare and apply this profoundly nourishing hair treatment.

Why Castor Oil and Banana Make the Perfect Hair Conditioner

Castor Oil: The Moisture-Rich Hair Healer

- **Deep Moisturization:** Castor oil is known for its thick, rich consistency. Thus, it deeply penetrates the hair shaft and locks moisture. It will, therefore, be very helpful if the hair is dry, damaged, or brittle. Because castor oil forms a barrier on the hair strands, moisture is not allowed to escape, keeping the hair hydrated and supple.

- **Promotes Hair Growth:** Castor oil contains a high quantity of ricinoleic acid, a type of fatty acid that increases blood flow to the scalp, thereby stimulating hair follicles and improving hair growth. Continuous application can result in noticeable full and thick hair.

- **Strengthens Hair:** This oil nourishes the hair by fortifying the shaft to prevent breakage and split ends. In fact, as time goes on, hair becomes stronger and more resistant to further breakdown caused by styling techniques and environmental stressors.

- **Adds Shine and Smoothness:** Castor oil's emollient properties smooth the cuticle of the hair, reducing frizz. The hair will be easy to manage and style, and it will have a natural, healthy shine and a silky, soft finish.

Banana: The Natural Hair Softener

- **Rich in Vitamins and Minerals:** Rich in nutritional value, bananas contain an impressive mixture of vitamins A, B6, C, and E and potassium, which are all essential elements for maintaining good hair.

These nutrients help strengthen the hair, avoid breakage, and generally promote healthy hair.

- **Improves Elasticity:** The vitamins and natural oils in bananas feed hair elasticity, which in turn prevents hair from breaking easily and getting damaged. This works perfectly for people who have dry or brittle hair, as it maintains their hair's strength and elasticity.

- **Moisturizes and Hydrates:** Bananas also naturally moisten and give intense hydration to the hair and scalp. That is why it is an excellent ingredient in fighting dryness or any moisture imbalance within the hair.

- **Adds Natural Shine:** The natural sugars in bananas help lock moisture, adding a nice sheen to the hair. When mixed with castor oil, bananas will make your hair look far more wholesome overall.

Benefits of the Castor Oil and Banana Hair Conditioner

Deep Conditioning and Hydration

- **Restores Moisture Balance:** This conditioner deeply moisturizes the hair to restore moisture balance to dry, damaged strands. Castor oil and banana will help inject essential nutrients and moisture into your hair, leaving it soft, smooth, and manageable.

- **Prevents and Repairs Damage:** The nourishing rich properties of castor oil and banana repair the existing breakage and help prevent further damage. Strengthening the hair shaft and improving elasticity, this conditioner prevents split ends and hair breakage, hence promoting healthy hair growth.

Enhances Hair Growth and Thickness

- **Stimulates Scalp Circulation:** Castor oil helps improve blood circulation to the scalp, stimulating hair follicles for hair growth and increasing hair density. This conditioner will continuously provide you with thicker and fuller hair.
- **Nourishes Hair Follicles:** Bananas are rich in vitamins and minerals, which help nourish hair follicles, promoting healthy hair growth and preventing hair loss. This is the ideal conditioner for anyone looking for natural ways to enhance hair growth.

Improves Hair Texture and Appearance

- **Adds Shine and Luster:** Since bananas contain natural oil and sugar, mixing them with smoothing castor oil adds a beautiful, natural shine to the hair. This conditioner improves the overall appearance of your hair, making it appear healthier and more vibrant.
- **Reduces Frizz and Tangles:** Castor oil's emollient properties smooth the hair cuticle, reducing frizz. It is also easier to detangle or style. All this leaves your hair feeling silky and soft with a smooth, polished finish.

How to Make the Castor Oil and Banana Hair Conditioner

Ingredients:

- 2 tablespoons of castor oil (cold-pressed and hexane-free)
- 1 ripe banana (organic if possible)
- 1 tablespoon of honey (optional, for added moisture and shine)
- 1 tablespoon of coconut oil (optional, for extra nourishment)
- A few drops of essential oil (such as lavender or rosemary, optional for fragrance and scalp health)

Instructions:

- Prepare the Banana: Peel the overripe banana and cut it into small pieces. Place the cut pieces in a blender or food processor until they are well blended, resulting in a smooth, no-lump puree. This is really important for even banana distribution in your hair and for avoiding chunks falling off everywhere.
- Mix the Oils: Mix the castor oil and coconut oil in a small bowl. If desired, gently warm by setting the bowl into another bowl filled with hot water. This will help mix better and ensure even distribution throughout the conditioner.
- Combine Ingredients: Add the banana puree and honey to the oil mixture. Mix until all the ingredients are well combined into a smooth, creamy paste. If desired, add a few drops of your favorite essential oil, as these will not only give fragrance but also benefit the scalp.

- Application: First, take your clean and damp hair and section it out so that the conditioner is evenly distributed. Apply generously from the roots down to the tips of your hair. Please use a wide-tooth comb to help coat it evenly and detangle it.
- Let It Sit: Once your hair is fully coated, put it under a shower cap or into a warm towel for better penetration of the conditioner deep within the shafts of the hair. Leave the conditioner in for 20-30 minutes to allow time for the nutrients to absorb.
- Rinse Thoroughly: After the conditioning time has passed, rinse your hair with warm water until all signs of conditioner are washed out. Rinse well so that no build-up or residue weighing remains on your hair.
- Style as Usual: After rinsing, you can style your hair as usual. For best results, allow your hair to air dry, preserving the moisture and nutrients from the conditioner.

Tips for Maximum Benefits

Frequency of Use

- **For Dry or Damaged Hair:** Use the Castor Oil and Banana Hair Conditioner once a week to restore moisture, repair damage, and maintain hair health.
- **For Normal Hair:** Use the conditioner once every two weeks to keep your hair nourished and shiny without over-conditioning.

Customize Your Conditioner

- **For Oily Hair:** For oily hair, use less castor oil and apply it only at the end of the hair, avoiding the scalp.

- **For Extra Frizz Control:** Add a teaspoon of aloe vera gel to the conditioner for added frizz-fighting and more moisture.
- **For Intense Repair:** If your hair is severely damaged, add an egg yolk to the above mixture. The egg's proteins will help strengthen and repair the hair shaft.

Storage

- Because this conditioner contains fresh banana, it is best used fresh. If you have some leftovers, you can store the mixture in an airtight container in the refrigerator for as long as 24 hours. Bring the conditioner to room temperature before reapplying.

Avoid Overloading Your Hair

- It's a really nourishing conditioner, but overused or too frequently it has the potential to weigh hair down. Use sparingly and make sure to scale back frequency depending on your hair's needs.

The Castor Oil and Banana Hair Conditioner is a sumptuous, nutrient-based treatment that transforms dry and damaged hair into silky, shiny, and full of life. This conditioner leverages the moisturizing effect of castor oil and the nourishment of banana for deep moisturizing, strengthening the hair shaft, and amplifying shine naturally. Whether your locks suffer from environmental damage or heat styling or need that extra special TLC, this natural conditioner is a powerhouse in your hair care arsenal.

When used regularly, this conditioner can provide various benefits: healthier hair that is resistant to environmental influences and will appear as good as it feels. Your hair will become strong, soft, and manageable and give an overall shine of health and vitality. Harness the power of nature and put your hair in its natural position with the Castor Oil and Banana Hair Conditioner.

Castor Oil and Egg Protein Hair Mask: A Strengthening and Nourishing Treatment for Resilient Hair

Hair can inherit stress from the environment, styling, coloring, and general wear and tear. In time, this makes the hair weak and brittle, prone to breakage, split ends, and generally damaged. To restore or maintain your hair's strength and health, one must rely on natural remedies, such as the Castor Oil and Egg Protein Hair Mask. It provides an effective combination of castor oil and egg that deeply nourishes, hydrates, and replenishes vital proteins within the hair to repair damage, strengthen the hair shaft, and promote healthy hair growth. Herein, we look at how using castor oil and egg as a hair mask together can be effective, as well as the preparation and application, and take a few tips here on maximizing the benefits.

Why Castor Oil and Egg Make a Powerful Hair Mask

Castor Oil: The Ultimate Moisturizer and Growth Stimulator

- **Deep Moisturization:** Castor oil is rich in fatty acids, primarily ricinoleic acid, a substance responsible for deeply nourishing the hair into the hair shaft and scalp. The thickness and viscosity of castor oil enable this oil to penetrate deep into the hair shaft by locking moisture inside and forming protection against environmental damage to the hair.

- **Promotes Hair Growth:** Castor oil may help stimulate hair growth because of its enhancing action on the blood circulation to the scalp, which keeps the hair follicles healthy. Regular application of this oil makes hair thick and strong, thus making it very difficult for hair to fall and promote growth.

- **Strengthens and Protects:** The nutrients in castor oil strengthen the hair shaft, making it harder to break or even split. This protective effect helps the hair be strong and not easily damaged by style, heat, or environmental elements.

Egg: A Natural Protein Powerhouse

- **Rich in Proteins:** Eggs are a correct source of high-quality proteins, which help build hair strength and structure. Proteins in eggs help repair and rebuild damaged hair, restoring elasticity and preventing breakages.

- **Vitamins and Minerals:** Eggs contain all different types of vitamins, including biotin, which is helpful for the health of your hair. Biotin adds extra strength to your hair while minimizing hair loss and positively stimulates hair growth. Eggs also contain essential minerals such as sulfur that will support keratin production, a necessary protein for the hair.

- **Adds Shine and Softness:** The nutrients within the egg help to smoothen the cuticle of the hair, adding a natural shine and softness. This makes the hair easier to manage and style, giving it a healthy, lustrous look.

Benefits of the Castor Oil and Egg Protein Hair Mask

Strengthens and Repairs Damaged Hair

- Rebuilds Hair Structure: The proteins in eggs repair damaged hair by filling in gaps and cracks along the shaft, essentially restoring it to its natural structure and strength. This reduces the risk of breakage and split ends, leading to much healthier and more resilient hair.
- Fortifies the Hair Shaft: The oil acts as a nutritious agent that strengthens the hair shaft, helping it prevent breakage and proving much stronger. Combining these properties with the protein-enriched properties of eggs can create an intense treatment through this hair mask, strengthening hair from the inside out.

Promotes Hair Growth and Reduces Hair Loss

- **Stimulates Hair Follicles:** Because castor oil facilitates an increase in blood flow to the scalp, it stimulates the hair follicles and encourages the growth of new hair. Eggs also help nourish the follicle further, providing nutrients for healthy hair growth and minimizing hair loss.
- **Prevents Hair Thinning:** If applied regularly, this hair mask can prevent hair thinning. It strengthens the hair shaft and encourages the growth of more intense hair, making it an excellent treatment for people with hair loss or thinning.

Enhances Hair Texture and Appearance

Adds Shine and Smoothness: The moisturizing action of castor oil, combined with the smoothing action of egg proteins, helps improve your hair's general aspect and texture. This hair mask will leave hair soft, smooth, and shiny-looking, with a healthy, vibrant look.

Improves Manageability: This mask rehydrates hair with moisture and strength, making it more manageable and accessible to style. Frizz, tangles, and flyaways are minimized, providing smoother, more controlled hair that is easier to work with.

How to Make the Castor Oil and Egg Protein Hair Mask

Ingredients:

- 2 tablespoons of castor oil (cold-pressed and hexane-free)
- 1 large egg (organic if possible)
- 1 tablespoon of olive oil or coconut oil (optional, for added moisture)
- A few drops of essential oil (such as rosemary or lavender, optional for fragrance and scalp health)

Instructions:

- **Prepare the Egg:** Crack the egg into a small bowl and beat it lightly with a fork until the yolk and white are thoroughly combined. Eggs can be used whole for normal hair, just the yolk for dry hair, or just the white for oily hair.
- **Mix the Oils:** In a separate bowl, add the castor oil mixed with olive or coconut oil. Both these oils add

more moisture and nourishment to the mask, making it even better for applying to dry or damaged hair.

- **Combine the Ingredients:** Progressively add the beaten egg to the oil mixture, stirring continuously to ensure the ingredients mix well. It should be smooth, creamy, and free of lumps.

- **Application:** Make sure hair is washed and damp before application. Part the hair into sections for even application of the mask. Generously apply at the roots and work down to the ends with a wide-toothed comb for even distribution without tangling.

- **Let It Sit:** Once the mask has been completely applied, cover your hair with a shower cap or a heated towel to help the product penetrate the hair shaft deeply. Leave the mask on for 20-30 minutes so the nutrients can fully be absorbed.

- **Rinse Thoroughly:** After the conditioning time, shampoo your hair with cold or lukewarm water to remove all mask traces. Avoid hot water at this moment, as it will cook the egg and leave its residue in your hair.

- **Condition as Usual:** After rinsing out the mask, follow up with a light conditioner to seal the moisture and smooth the hair cuticle. You can also use a leave-in conditioner or a few drops of castor oil to add shine and protection.

Tips for Maximum Benefits

Frequency of Use

- For Damaged or Dry Hair: Use the Castor Oil and Egg Protein Hair Mask once a week to repair damage, strengthen hair, and restore moisture.

- For Normal Hair: Use the mask once every two weeks to maintain hair health and prevent damage.

Customize Your Mask

- For Oily Hair: If your hair is oily, use only the white of the egg and reduce the amount of castor oil. You can add a few drops of lemon juice to control excess oiliness and maintain a better scalp balance.
- For Extra Moisture: Add a tablespoon of honey or yogurt to the mask for extra hydration. Honey is a natural humectant that helps lock moisture in, while yogurt adds extra proteins and probiotics to nourish the scalp.

Avoid Overloading Your Hair

- While this mask is very helpful, it can be overused too much or too often. It will weigh your hair down, especially for those with finer hair. Adjust accordingly based on how your hair responds to this treatment.

Storage

- This mask is best used fresh since it contains fresh ingredients. If the mixture is left over, it may be stored in an airtight container in the refrigerator for 24 hours. Bring the mask to room temperature before applying it.

Rinsing and Finishing

- Make sure to rinse out the mask thoroughly with cool or lukewarm water so you don't end up cooking the egg in your hair. After this, allow your hair to air dry if possible, as this helps to lock in the moisture and nutrients from the mask.

Castor Oil and Egg Protein Hair Mask is an extremely powerful natural treatment for hair, helping to strengthen, nourish, and rejuvenate it. This hair mask combines deep moisturizing action with the protein-enriched nourishment of eggs to give your hair all it needs to stay healthy, strong, and vibrant. Whether damaged, dry, or needing a boost, this mask will restore your hair's natural beauty and resilience.

In fact, this hair mask should greatly improve hair strength, texture, and appearance. Through the regular application, you can get stronger, softer hair that's easier to manage, has a natural sheen and reflects its health. So, step into the benefits of this natural remedy and get ready to give your hair what it deserves with the Castor Oil and Egg Protein Hair Mask.

Castor Oil and Rosemary Brow Booster: A Natural Formula for Fuller, Healthier Eyebrows

The eyebrow is essential in giving a frame to the face and adding to one's appearance. Though complete, well-defined brows have become a beauty staple, nobody has thick eyebrows. Over-plucking can make your eyebrows thin or sometimes sparse due to hormonal changes and aging, which require daily filling with makeup. However, with the right natural ingredients, it is without doubt that you can encourage fuller and healthier eyebrow growth. Both castor oil and rosemary essential oil are potent, natural boosters of brow growth-strengthening hair follicles for fuller, thicker eyebrows. We shall cover the benefits of using castor oil with rosemary, teach you how to make your brow booster, and give you some tips on how to get the most out of this recipe.

Why Castor Oil and Rosemary Are the Perfect Brow Booster

Castor Oil: The Ultimate Growth and Strengthening Agent

- **Nutrient-Rich Composition:** Castor oil contains essential fatty acids, most prevalently ricinoleic acid, an active complex responsible for moisturizing, nourishing, and performing anti-inflammatory actions. These constituents play the most crucial role in hair growth and scalp health.
- **Promotes Hair Growth:** Castor oil has traditionally been used to increase hair growth. This is because it efficiently enhances blood flow into the hair follicles, which receive increased oxygenation and nourishment, yielding thicker and fuller eyebrows.
- **Strengthens Hair Follicles:** Castor oil moisturizes and, therefore, helps strengthen the existing brow hairs, making them less prone to breakage and fallout. This helps maintain the integrity of your brows while they grow thicker and healthier.

Rosemary Essential Oil: A Powerful Hair Growth Stimulant

- **Improves Circulation:** Rosemary essential oil is known to promote blood flow when applied topically. Increased blood flow around the brow will ensure that hair follicles receive adequate nutrition for developing new brow hairs.

- **Strengthens Hair Roots:** Rosemary oil is fully loaded with antioxidants, effectively rescuing hair follicles from damage caused by free radicals and other environmental stressors. This firms the hair's roots, reducing every chance of brow hair loss.
- **Balances Oil Production:** Rosemary oil normalizes sebum production in the brow area, which is essential for maintaining favorable hair growth conditions. This prevents greasiness or dryness in the area where the eyebrows are found; either extreme can inhibit hair growth.

Benefits of the Castor Oil and Rosemary Brow Booster

Promotes Fuller, Thicker Eyebrows

- **Stimulates Hair Follicles:** This combination of castor oil and rosemary essential oil synergistically stimulates the hair follicles in the brow area to promote new growth. Consistently using it will give you complete, thicker brows that require less makeup and maintenance.
- **Reduces Brow Hair Loss:** This brow booster nourishes and strengthens your hair follicles to minimize hair loss, enabling you to retain more natural brow hairs as they grow.

Strengthens and Conditions Existing Brow Hairs

- **Prevents Breakage:** This forms a deep moisturizing, strengthening, and preventing breakage or fallout of brow hairs. The effect is that the brows are fuller, healthier, and more resilient.
- **Conditions the Brow Area:** Applying castor oil and rosemary oil will help condition the skin around the

brows and prevent dryness and flakiness. It produces a healthy environment in which brows grow continuously.

Natural, Safe, and Easy to Use

- **Free from Harsh Chemicals:** Unlike many other commercial brow-growing products, which contain synthetically produced active ingredients and potentially harsh chemicals, this Castor Oil and Rosemary Brow Booster is all-natural and, thus, absolutely safe for everyday use. It's highly suitable for people with sensitive skin or wanting to avoid chemical-based beauty products.
- **Easy Application:** This brow booster is pretty easy to make and apply, so it won't be complicated for one to fit into their everyday beauty routines. It will take only a few minutes daily, and over time, it will help support your eyebrows to be healthier and fuller.

How to Make the Castor Oil and Rosemary Brow Booster

Ingredients:

- 1 tablespoon of castor oil (cold-pressed and hexane-free)
- 2-3 drops of rosemary essential oil
- A clean mascara wand or a spoolie brush for application
- A small, clean container with a lid for storage

Instructions:

- **Combine the Ingredients:** In a small, clean container, combine 1 tablespoon of the castor oil with 2-3 drops of rosemary essential oil. Stir well to ensure the mixture is incorporated correctly.

- **Store Properly:** Once mixed, place the brow booster in a container with a tight lid to avoid exposing it to air and light, which can degrade the essential oils.

Application:

- **Brow preparation:** Before applying the brow booster, your eyebrows should be fresh and free of makeup or skincare products.
- Insert a clean mascara wand or a spoolie brush into the mixture, removing the excess oil so it doesn't drip.
- Apply the oil mixture lightly onto your eyebrows, working from the roots and covering each hair in your brow.
- Brush it through your brows with the brush so the oil gets equally distributed.
- **Let It Absorb:** Leave the brow booster overnight to allow the oils to reach the root of the hair follicles and skin. After soaking in for several hours, the residual oil can be removed by washing the face in the morning.

Daily Use: Repeat this every night before bed, and you will have healthier, fuller brows over time.

Tips for Maximizing Results

Be Consistent

- Consistency is key to hair growth. Using the Castor Oil and Rosemary Brow Booster daily, preferably at night, give your brows the best chance of growing strong over time.

Massage the Brow Area

- Massage the brow area gently for a minute or two after application to increase the effect of this brow booster. The massage will stimulate blood flow and help the oils penetrate deep into the hair follicle.

Pair with a Healthy Diet

- Your diet is crucial for the health of your hair, and obviously, this includes your eyebrows as well. Ensure that you are consuming sufficient amounts of nutrients such as vitamins and minerals, especially biotin, Vitamin E, and Omega-3, which are responsible for the growth and strengthening of your hair.

Avoid Over-Plucking

- Don't over-pluck or wax your brows if you're trying to grow them. This will give the brow booster the best chance of working well. If you have to shape your eyebrows, do so minimally and with caution.

Patch Test Before Use

- Rosemary essential oil is very strong, so it is not recommended to apply the brow booster to your eyebrows without a patch test. You can apply the mixture to a small and less visible skin area and leave it for 24 hours to see if irritation occurs. If it doesn't, you can safely use the product for your brows.

For people who want fuller, healthier eyebrows, the Castor Oil and Rosemary Brow Booster is as simple as it is effective. "By feeding hair growth with this treatment, castor oil, and rosemary essential oil will help nourish hair follicles, strengthen existing brow hairs, and even spur new growth, thus creating thicker and fuller brows.

This brow booster naturally and effectively works against sparse eyebrows without using chemical-based products or invasive procedures. When applied regularly, it will make notable improvements concerning the fullness and health of your brows, allowing you to manage a more polished, younger look.

Let nature's marvels work magic for you with Castor Oil and Rosemary Brow Booster- a simple yet power-packed way to end the brow game and get the bold and beautiful brows you always wanted.

By following these safety tips, readers will be able to confidently add castor oil to their beauty routine and ensure that any adverse effects will be avoided and an excellent experience.

In Chapter 3 we discussed in detail the many ways one can use castor oil when making various natural beauty products. It is also used in a variety of recipes like lip balms and moisturizers. Adding other natural ingredients to such recipes creates personalized beauty solutions that are perfect and most ideal for particular needs. Since castor oil is compatible with a range of carrier oils, the possibilities for achieving optimal skin and hair health are virtually endless. With proper usage procedures, readers will be able to reap the complete benefits of castor oil without running any risk of its adverse side effects. Therefore, with this newfound knowledge, anyone can harness the power of castor oil in shiny hair and glowing skin, turning one's home into a paradise for natural beauty.

Part 2: Castor Oil for Health and Pain Relief

Chapter 4:
Castor Oil Relieves Pain, Heals Muscles and Joints

Castor oil has been an ally for soothing muscles and joints and also for cosmetic purposes. It is among the most powerful anti-inflammatory and pain relievers in natural medicine, hence perfect for arthritis patients, people with chronic joint pains, and muscle aches. This work will explain everything from muscular soreness to inflammation reduction in arthritic joints, while touching on a wide range of other pain management applications, from irregular menstrual cycles and ovarian cysts to arthritis and fibromyalgia, as well as injuries-sports or otherwise. The readers will be taken through the basic science that underlines why castor oil works, along with practical applications and motivational stories by people who have already experienced relief.

Natural Inflammation Reduction with Castor Oil for Arthritis and Joint Pain

Arthritis, by statistic counts, affects millions worldwide, caused by unending aching, stiffness, and swelling within the joints. While traditional therapies like medicine and physical therapy can offer some relief, many seek alternative remedies away from conventional methods using natural remedies such as castor oil. This is because ricinoleic acid is an effective anti-inflammatory compound found in this type of oil, which, upon topical application, permeates through the skin into the target tissues that are inflamed. This section covers how one can incorporate castor oil into an arthritis treatment regimen.

Anti-Inflammatory Properties: Ricinoleic acid is known to be an effective inhibitor of inflammation synthesis. Thus, this oil acts well deep inside skin tissue by reducing the pain of joints and swelling when applied at the site.

Pain Relief: Osteoarthritis is a form of arthritis caused by the degeneration of cartilage between bones. Since this degeneration leads to the friction of bone against bone, pain and stiffness are stimulated. Individuals with osteoarthritis may highly be able to find castor oil useful because large doses, taken frequently, lubricate the area of the joint, increasing mobility and lowering pain.

Application Method: Heat castor oil and massage it gently into the arthritic joints to relieve pain. Do this twice a day. For further relief, apply a castor oil pack, described later in this chapter, to the aching area.

Encouraging Cartilage Health: By improving circulation and reducing oxidative stress, two extremely important factors involved in maintaining healthy joints throughout the lifetime, castor oil may be effective in stimulating new growth of cartilage. Castor oil is not a cure for arthritis but can reduce the progression of arthritic symptoms over time.

Those with arthritis who use castor oil consistently report increased mobility, reduced pain, and a more organic and holistic response to inflammation.

How Castor Oil Can Ease and Heal Muscle Aches and Pains

Muscle aches and pains are often perceived by persons of all ages, whether through strenuous exercise or in most instances, through daily wear and tear. Castor oil has a soothing-warming effect to alleviate pain, relax contracted muscles, and accelerate the healing process. This section discusses some of the many muscle groups wherein castor oil can help ease pain.

Reducing Muscle Soreness: Muscle soreness is a result of lactic acid buildup and microtears in muscle fibers, post a high-intensity workout session or exercise. Castor oil helps eliminate lactic acid by releasing tensed muscles, thus speeding up the healing process, and enhancing blood flow.

Application: Soak warm castor oil into your palms and massage it onto those painful spots in circular motions. The warmth in the oil and light pressure may relieve pain and tension.

Relieving Muscle Cramps: Muscle cramps can be very painful and harassing. They are often caused by electrolyte imbalances and dehydration. Castor oil is effective in reducing the frequency and intensity of cramps due to its natural concentration of magnesium and its ability to hydrate deeply.

Following the application of castor oil to the cramping muscle, wrap the affected area with a warm cloth or heating pad for 20 minutes. This method allows for deeper penetration of the oil, thus offering quicker relief.

Recovery after Workout: Adding castor oil to their post-recovery treatment after a workout is another good way for athletes and fitness enthusiasts to experience its regenerative properties. The time between sets of exercises will be shorter, and the recovery time will also be less, as it will reduce inflammation and muscle strain.

Relax the massage of worked-out muscles with castor oil and a few drops of essential oils like eucalyptus or lavender. The application of castor oil is a natural alternative to over-the-counter pain medicines due to its relaxing and anti-inflammable nature, hence serving as a flexible cure for muscle-related ailments.

How to Use Castor Oil Wraps for Pain

Castor oil compresses or wraps are among the most effective ways to tap into its therapeutic properties for pain relief. For better absorption, a castor oil wrap can be used by dipping a cloth into hot castor oil, wrapping up the affected area, and heating it. This would work best on deeper pains, such as in the case of joint pain, muscle strains, and stomach aches. In the following, we will discuss how castor oil wraps are applied for various kinds of pains.

Mechanism of Action: The heat opens the pores and dilates the vessels to make more blood flow through. As a result, the ricinoleic acid will be more able to penetrate more into tissues. Besides this efficient delivery of the therapeutic agent, improved circulation will provide cleaning of impurities and toxins around the area in question.

Wraps for Joint Pain: Castor oil wraps work wonderfully for joint pains caused by arthritis. The anti-inflammation properties of the oil, along with the heat of the wrap, aid in soothing stiffness and swelling.

Directions: Wet a clean cotton towel with warm castor oil and apply it to the diseased joint. Wrap it with plastic wrap or a heating pad to keep it hot. Keep on for thirty to sixty minutes maximum.

Wrapping Castor Oil for Muscle Strains: Castor oil wraps can also be done in the case of muscle injuries or strains. The oil is a good option for athletes or individuals who have muscle injuries due to its anti-inflammatory characteristics that reduce healing time.

Instructions: Same as for treatment of joint pain. Allow the application to focus on the area of strained muscle. Do it two to three times a week until the discomfort is gone.

Wraps for stomach pain: Castor oil wraps can be used in addition to the relief of joint and muscular pain, including stomach pain resulting from bloating, constipation, or menstrual colic. Of the many benefits of castor oil, an increase in the circulation in the abdomen promotes pain relief and digestion.

Wrap the lower abdomen with the wrap. Leave on for 30 minutes, repeat as frequently as needed for relief.

Castor oil wraps are a great complement to any pain treatment. The major reason is that it offers a safe, non-invasive solution to the problems of chronic pain.

Success Stories: Real Changes in People's Lives

Castor oil pain relief has been sought and gained by many individuals, greatly enhancing their quality of life. This section provides direct accounts from persons who have successfully managed pain using castor oil. Success stories represent the effectiveness of castor oil in natural healing, from sportive individuals recuperating from muscular injuries to persons suffering from arthritis symptoms and finding relief from joint discomfort.

Anna's Story: Arthritis ease After decades of painkillers for her severe osteoarthritis of the knees and, at best, temporary relief, Anna, a 58-year-old woman began using castor oil wraps. Having used the wraps for several weeks on a regular basis, she found that she was becoming much more mobile with less discomfort; therefore, she was able to get back into doing a lot of things that not so long ago she had given up hope ever being able to do.

John's Experience with Recuperation After Exercise: John was a competitive runner who would constantly deal with injuries and muscle soreness. After he learned about rubbing down his muscles with castor oil, he began to use it after a session at the gym. He found that his recuperation time came quicker after a couple of weeks enabling him to push harder without the usual muscular soreness and fatigue.

Transformation of Sara: How to Deal with Menstrual Pain: All her life, Sara had to cope with a sharp cramp in her menstrual cycle. She would take medicines to try to survive the month. Castor oil wraps on the stomach reduced the pain and cramps that were being faced. Castor oil was her monthly remedy to get her out of prescription medication.

These testimonials provide evidence that, applied rightly, castor oil can indeed make a difference in the lives of people who suffer from chronic pain by offering them a harmless, easy, and natural alternative to traditional pain-relieving methods.

We have reviewed, within Chapter 4, the amazing benefits that castor oil delivers for pain relief, including how this herbal remedy may reduce inflammation, soothe pains within the muscles, and create persistent relief from pains in joints. Castor oil can be thought of as a natural alternative to conventional pain relievers for arthritis, among other painful disorders, and recovery after workouts. Castor oil has proved to be one of the most powerful tools for healing and pain relief, which may be employed in the form of direct applications, massage, or wraps. Centuries of use and research-supported advantages secure castor oil as one of nature's best treatments against joint and muscular pain.

Chapter 5:
Using Castor Oil for Natural Healing

Holistic health has grown in demand over the past few years as people seek natural remedies that promote well-being without the side effects observed with conventional treatment. Other than the analgesic and cosmetic properties, castor oil is also used for therapeutic purposes. Its complex composition and, in particular, the content of high ricinoleic acid promote deep and systemic healing in addition to superficial advantages. Castor oil is a vital tool for anyone trying to include natural remedies into his or her health regimen because it can do anything from enhancing digestion and immunity to cleansing the body. In this chapter, we will see how castor oil can help in detoxification, making your stomach strong, increasing your immunity level, and making functions of the liver and kidney more active.

Increasing Immunity with the Use of Castor Oil: The Benefits of Lymph

The immune system is the first line of defense of our body against diseases. The healthy functioning of the lymphatic system exerts a great influence on the effectiveness of the immune system. Though called the draining system of the body, it clears residues, toxins, and other unwanted elements from the tissues and organs. A slow or clogged lymphatic system can yield a weak immune system and several other health issues.

The castor oil treatment is a potent natural remedy that helps strengthen the immune system because it increases lymphatic stimulation.

Lymphatic Stimulation: Studies have revealed that the content of ricinoleic acid present in castor oil has a positive effect on lymphatic flow since it stimulates it, thereby aiding the body in easily removing its waste. In addition to the reduction of inflammation, a properly working lymphatic system also helps the body dispose of disease-causing pathogens with great efficiency.

Application: Castor oil packs are one of the most effective ways to promote lymphatic drainage. Castor oil applied topically enters the skin, thereby increasing lymph flow and, in effect, diminishes lymph congestion. To activate the immune function, apply a hot castor oil pack over the abdomen or lymphatic tissue sites such as the groin or underarms for 30 to 60 minutes.

Increased WBC Production: It has been shown that through the daily administration of castor oil, increased production of white blood cells is a necessity for immune protection. Through the action of castor oil, there is an effect of improved circulation and lymphatic flow, which results in increased action by the body's defense mechanisms.

Reduce Inflammation: Often, inflammation is simply a symptom of the immune system over-compensating for the presence of certain toxins or bacteria. Anti-inflammatory properties within the castor oil support immune system relaxation so that it's better able to focus on genuine threats rather than overreacting to stimuli that really aren't worthy of concern.

All told, when it comes to the use of castor oil as part of healthy lymphatic protocol, consistent use of the oil will lead to an optimized immune system, reduced incidence of disease, and a healthier lifestyle altogether.

Digestive Health Support: Using Castor Oil for Support in Digestion

Integrative well-being depends a great deal on gut health, which controls everything from mood to digestion. Constipation is a common issue that, if not resolved, brings uneasiness, bloating, and long-term effects on health. Classically used for natural laxative products, castor oil can be of great help for promoting regularity and keeping intestines healthy.

Natural Laxative Properties: One of the oldest and most well-recognized uses of castor oil is to provide relief from constipation. Upon ingestion, ricinoleic acid acts on the colon and small intestine to increase contractions of the muscles to move foods and other material along the digestive tract.

For Constipation: It acts as a purgative with 1-2 teaspoons of oral castor oil in a few hours. It is taken for better results on an empty stomach, and use is not intended to be frequent so as not to develop dependence.

Improved Digestion: Castor oil aids in overall digestion, other than its laxative effects. Promoting bowel regularity helps the body efficiently eliminate wastes and toxins, which is the basis of gut health.

Prevention of Gas and Bloating: Often, uncomfortable gas and bloating result from constipation. Castor oil prevents such symptoms coming from constipation and thus provides ease in digestion by promoting bowel movements that result in non-hardened stool.

Instead of artificial laxatives, castor oil offers a natural and safe solution that meets the needs of good gut health without disagreeable side effects associated with traditional prescription medications.

Castor Oil Packs Are Ideal For Promoting Detoxification Within Your Body System For It To Heal

Detoxification is vital in holistic health as it enables the body to clear any accumulated poisons, which could lead to disease. Castor oil is a very strong detoxifier; hence, it will be handy in cleaning and healing processes since it easily penetrates into the tissues.

How Castor Oil Detoxifies: The ability of castor oil to raise the levels of lymphatic and blood flow and to promote skin and alimentary canal excretion of toxins is what allows the oil to be described as a detoxifying agent. Castor oil stimulates these cleansing processes, which in turn help the body dispose of toxic waste and improve general health and vitality.

Detoxification with Castor Oil Packs: Among all the usages of castor oil, detoxification is definitely one of the most effective ways. Applying a pack of castor oil on the belly may activate the organs responsible for detoxification, such as the liver, kidneys, and intestines.

Instructions for the Castor Oil Pack: After dipping a clean cloth in hot castor oil, place it on the abdomen and allow it to stay there for thirty to sixty minutes assisted by a heating pad or plastic wrap. This procedure enables the oil to penetrate deep into the tissues, which supersedes the cleansing process, leaving a healing feeling.

Removing Toxins Through the Skin: With its unique property to penetrate through the skin, castor oil helps eliminate toxins from deeper layers of tissues. Besides such several physical benefits, a castor oil pack encourages your body to get rid of all kinds of wastes and metabolic by-products, which will leave you with feelings of lightness and energy.

Castor oil packs can be part of the way to help you increase your energy, and general sense of well-being, and support improved digestion through the course of detoxification.

Renal and Hepatic Support: The Missing Link in Detoxification

The main detoxification organs are the liver and kidneys, which help purify the blood, thereby keeping the body healthy. In talking detoxification, one of the most important yet influential substances on proper functioning is castor oil, which promotes the functioning of such vital organs.

Liver Support: The liver is responsible for breaking down and eliminating blood toxins through the body. Castor oil supports the liver through the enhancement of its detoxification capability in the body and by stimulating liver activity. Bile is an important compound in the digestion and elimination of toxins, and production may be stimulated through regular application of castor oil packs to the liver area.

Application: Two times a week, apply a warm castor oil pack to the liver - located on the right side of the abdomen just below the level of the lower ribs - for thirty to sixty minutes. In particular, this can be effective in stimulating liver activity in individuals whose liver may be sluggish as a result of nutritional deficiencies and/or environmental toxins.

Supporting the Kidneys: Your kidneys serve to filter waste products out of your blood and eliminate those wastes and excesses while maintaining fluid balance within your body. Castor oil serves to support the kidneys in their detoxifying function by reducing inflammation and increasing blood flow to them.

How to apply: Apply a castor oil pack to the area of the lower back that houses the kidneys. This will support great improvements to the health of your kidneys, as it reduces inflammation and increases circulation.

Supporting Detoxification Pathways: Castor oil becomes an effective detoxification support owing to the functions it operates on, including the kidney and liver. With support from the liver and kidneys, castor oil ensures optimum performance of the body's major detoxification pathways.

Added to a proper detoxification plan, the possible general improvement in health from this basic detox aid increased, as would be the reduced burden of health effects from the overaccumulation of toxins and delayed onset of chronic disease related to toxic overload.

For example, in Chapter 5, we discussed how castor oil has played an important role in holistic health and cited many applications beyond cosmetics and surface-level healing. Improved liver and kidney function, cleansing, immune stimulation, and supporting the gut are just a few of the applications that make castor oil a staple therapeutic agent in holistic health. Castor oil is good for anyone desiring improved general health, as it can stir the lymphatic system, enhance circulation, and help the body flush out toxins. With decades of effective use behind them, castor oil packs or their traditional form offer a myriad of benefits.

Castor Oil for Sleep Aid: A Natural Remedy for Restful Nights

First and foremost, a good night's sleep is chief among life's necessities, particularly for health and wellness. Too many of us, though, are not getting a whole night's rest because of our insomnia keeping us up or just not being able to sleep from all the stresses, anxieties, and other problems that abound. There are multitudes of over-the-counter and prescription aids for sleep; the catch to most of those usually includes side effects and addictive potential. Those seeking help from nature can try castor oil as a mild yet effective way of sleeping better. In fact, soothing and anti-inflammatory are the primary healing attributes of this plant derivative that eventually help the mind and body be in a restful sleeping stage. In this section, we talk about castor oil being used as an advantage for sleeping purposes, how it works, and ways to practically apply the extract to one's nighttime routine.

Why Castor Oil Is Effective as a Sleep Aid

Natural Relaxant

- **Soothing Properties:** Castor oil is concentrated with ricinoleic acid, a potent natural anti-inflammatory and analgesic. Topically, castor oil relieves muscle tension and pain and relaxes the body's combined factors to get someone into a restful sleep.

- **Calming the Nervous System:** Castor oil applied topically relaxes the nervous system. Its anxiolytic and stress-reducing properties help the mind ease into sleep more easily throughout the night.

Promotes Circulation

- **Improved Blood Flow:** One of the most well-known benefits associated with castor oil is its ability to promote blood flow to the skin. Increased blood flow can warm the body and provide a soothing sensation, making falling asleep easier.
- **Reducing Inflammation:** Castor oil may ease conditions that disrupt sleep, such as joint pain and other discomforts, by promoting circulation and reducing inflammation.

Supports Hormonal Balance

- **Regulating Sleep Hormones:** Castor oil has also played a role in supporting hormonal balance, a condition necessary for regulating sleep patterns. By supporting the production of hormones involved in regulating sleep, like cortisol and melatonin, castor oil may contribute to more consistent and restful sleep.

Gentle Detoxification

- **Cleansing the Body:** Castor oil has been known to possess detoxifying properties, mainly when applied as castor oil packs. The stimulating effect for removing toxins encourages a general detoxification process within the body, relieving the liver and digestive system from stress that may be prohibitive to improved health and sleep.

- **Improving Digestion:** A sound digestive system ensures a proper sleep pattern. Castor oil can aid digestion by reducing inflammation, regulating bowel habits, and alleviating discomfort that interferes with a good night's sleep.

Benefits of Using Castor Oil for Sleep

Enhances Sleep Quality

- **Deeper, More Restful Sleep:** Castor oil enhances sleep by relaxing the body and reducing pain. Users who apply it at bedtime confirm a deeper, more restorative sleep and also feel fresh the following day.
- **Reduces Sleep Disturbances:** Castor oil's soothing effect is an excellent antidote to sleep disturbances due to pain, stress, or anxiety. In other words, it means fewer nighttime interruptions and more constant sleep.

Eases Sleep-Related Discomfort

- **Relieves Muscle Tension and Pain:** Castor oil provides needed relief for those with muscle tension and pain that disturb sleeping. Because of its anti-inflammatory and analgesic properties, it may relax muscles and reduce pain, thus helping one sleep better and for longer periods.
- **Reduces Anxiety and Stress:** When used topically, castor oil may help relax the mind and lower anxiety and stress that interfere with night sleeping.

Supports Overall Well-Being

- **Promotes Detoxification:** On the other hand, regular consumption of castor oil aids in the body's detoxification process. This helps maintain overall health, and with a sounder body, one gets better rest and sleeps more regularly.
- **Balances Hormones:** Castor oil helps regulate sleep/wake patterns by normalizing hormonal processes, improving sleep quality.

How to Use Castor Oil for Sleep Aid

Castor Oil Pack for Relaxation

Ingredients:

- 1-2 tablespoons of castor oil (cold-pressed and hexane-free)
- A clean piece of flannel or cotton cloth
- Plastic wrap or a plastic sheet
- A heating pad or hot water bottle

Instructions:

- **Prepare the Castor Oil Pack:** Fold the flannel or cotton cloth into several layers and soak it in castor oil until saturated. The cloth should be large enough to cover the area of your body where you plan to apply the pack, such as your abdomen, lower back, or joints.
- **Apply the Pack:** Now, place the soaked cloth on the desired area of your body. Cover the cloth with plastic wrap to protect your clothing and bedding. Over the pack, one may apply a heating pad or hot

water bottle, which helps the oil absorb into the skin and relax the individual.

- **Relax and Rest:** Lie down in a comfortable position and relax, allowing the castor oil pack to do its work for 30-60 minutes. This is a beautiful time to practice deep breathing or meditation to enhance your relaxation process further.
- **Remove and Cleanse:** Following the treatment, remove the pack and cleanse with warm water or a mild soap to remove the residual oil. Then, store the cloth in a plastic bag for use later—castor oil packs may be reused numerous times before renewal is required.

Usage Tips:

- Use the castor oil pack 2-3 times a week, or as needed, to promote relaxation and improve sleep quality.
- For best results, use the pack in the evening before bedtime to help prepare your body for sleep.

Castor Oil Foot Massage

Ingredients:

- 1-2 teaspoons of castor oil (cold-pressed and hexane-free)
- A pair of cotton socks

Instructions:

- **Warm the Oil:** Warm the castor oil by placing the bottle in a bowl of hot water for a few minutes. This helps with better absorption and is also very soothing to massage.

- **Massage Your Feet:** Massage warm castor oil into your soles at bedtime, paying special attention to the arch and area around your toes. The feet contain many nerve endings and pressure points; hence, massaging them is one surefire way of relaxing.
- **Wear Socks:** After massaging the oil into your feet, slip on a pair of cotton socks to hold the oil in place and prevent the oil from staining your sheets.
- **Rest and Relax:** Lie down and relax while letting the castor oil absorb in. It will help soothe your nervous system, giving you that restful state required for falling asleep.

Usage Tips:

- Practice this massage technique nightly before bed to help you relax and improve your sleeping condition.
- If you find the smell of castor oil too overwhelming, mix a few drops of any calming essential oil-like lavender or chamomile-into the castor oil before massaging.

Castor Oil Scalp Treatment

Ingredients:

- 1 tablespoon of castor oil (cold-pressed and hexane-free)
- A few drops of lavender or chamomile essential oil (optional)

Instructions:

- **Mix the Oils:** Mix the castor oil with a few drops of your favorite essential oil in a small bowl. Lavender and chamomile have relaxing properties and are known to help induce good sleeping.
- **Massage the Scalp:** At night and before retiring to bed, massage your scalp with your fingertips in circular motions using gentle pressure, focusing more on the temples and the back of the neck.
- **Relax and Sleep:** Leave the oil on your scalp overnight to work its magic. The massage will relieve tension, which in turn relaxes you and allows you to fall asleep more easily.
- **Wash in the Morning:** In the morning, wash your hair as you normally would to remove the oil.

Usage Tips:

- Use this scalp treatment once or twice a week or whenever you need an extra boost of relaxation before bed.
- You can also enhance the relaxation effect by playing soothing music or deep breathing while rubbing your scalp.

Additional Tips for Better Sleep with Castor Oil

Establish a Relaxing Bedtime Routine

- Combining castor oil into one's nightly bedtime routine can help promote better sleep. You could try using castor oil in addition to any other relaxing nighttime routine, such as reading, meditation, or even taking a hot bath, to tell the body it is time to sleep.

Practice Deep Breathing

- Deep breathing exercises while applying castor oil or using a castor oil pack can further promote relaxation. Deep breathing relaxes the nervous system, calms stress and prepares the body for sleep.

Create a Sleep-Conducive Environment

- **Sleep-friendly bedroom:** Keep the bedroom calm, dark, and quiet. If necessary, use blackout curtains, earplugs, or a white noise machine. A comfortable mattress and pillows will also help you sleep well.

Stay Hydrated, but Not Too Close to Bedtime

- **Hydration is important;** however, it is best to avoid drinking a great deal of liquid prior to retiring for the night to avoid waking up to use the bathroom. The more you focus on water throughout your day, the fewer fluids are needed within the hour of bedtime.

Castor oil is one of those few all-purpose, strong natural remedies that can help improve the quality of sleep in several ways. Whether it is insomnia, poor sleep at night, or a sick feeling after a long day, these diverse applications of castor oil before bed can help one achieve more quality, restorative sleep. Here are some of the methods to apply castor oil for sleeping: from castor oil packs to foot massages and scalp treatments that will bring other benefits one may need.

Adding castor oil to one's bedtime routine allows the soothing and calming action of castor oil to positively affect the creation of a more restorative sleep environment. In due time, you will realize that you finally fell asleep, slept longer, and woke up fresh, renewed, and revitalized. Use Castor Oil as a natural sleep aid and leap toward overall health and wellness.

Stress-Relieving Bath Blends

In today's fast-paced world, stress is common and has become a part of each person's lifestyle, making every single side of life mentally and physically stressful. One way to release stress is to take a very luxurious and comfortable bath. The warm bath relaxes tired muscles and gives a relaxing effect and serenity to the natural ingredients such as essential oils, herbs, and castor oil. The tub could create more of a therapeutic experience, one experience – one that has much in common with a ritual in which one unwinds and then recharges. This section explores five stress-relieving bath blends using castor oil with calming essential oils and herbs, including soothing lavender & castor oil bath soak, tranquil eucalyptus & castor embrace bath elixir, calm chamomile & castor bath bedtime, peaceful peppermint & castor oil bath mixture, and rejuvenating lemongrass & castor oil blend.

Soothing Lavender & Castor Oil Bath Soak

Why It Works

It is one of the most popular essential oils for sleep and stress relief. Lavender oil is often credited for its calming and soothing effects, which can help one sleep with less anxiety while cooling down the nervous system. A bath soak is an especially critical tool when castor oil is applied deeply, moisturizes, softens the skin, and cools it down. Benefits.

Benefits

- **Calms the Mind and Body:** Lavender oil's calming scent helps to relax the mind and body, making it easier to let go of stress and tension.
- **Promotes Better Sleep:** A bath in lavender before retiring can contribute to better and deeper sleep due to reduced anxiety, and it helps the body prepare for rest.
- **Nourishes the Skin:** Castor oil is rich in moisturizing properties and gives skin hydration that leaves the skin soft, supple, and glowing after the bath.

How to Make and Use the Soothing Lavender & Castor Oil Bath Soak

Ingredients:

- 1/4 cup of castor oil (cold-pressed and hexane-free)
- 10-15 drops of lavender essential oil
- 1 cup of Epsom salts (optional, for additional muscle relaxation)
- Dried lavender buds (optional, for added fragrance and aesthetic appeal)
- A small jar or container for mixing

Instructions:

- **Combine the Ingredients:** Use a small jar or container to mix the castor oil with the lavender essential oil. If applicable, add the Epsom salts and dried lavender buds. Stir to combine everything well.

- **Prepare the Bath:** Fill your tub with warm water. As it fills, pour the mixture into the water, gently stirring with your hand to help the oil and salts disperse.
- **Soak and Relax:** Fill the tub with water to your liking, slide in, and soak for 20-30 minutes as you let the subtle aroma of lavender calm both body and mind, along with the hydrating feel of castor oil.
- **Rinse and Moisturize:** After soaking in the bath, use warm water to remove as much remaining oil from the skin as possible. Then, gently pat your skin dry and apply a light moisturizer if needed.

Usage Tips:

- Use this bath soak in the evening to help unwind after a long day or to promote better sleep.
- Store any leftover mixture in a cool, dark place, and shake well before each use.

Tranquil Eucalyptus & Castor Embrace Bath Elixir

Why It Works

Eucalyptus oil is famous for its refreshing and invigorating aroma. It promotes a clear mind and encourages deep breathing. It is particularly effective in respiratory problems, muscle strain, and mental fatigue. Mixed with castor oil in this bath elixir, it relaxes the body and renews the mind, thereby becoming ideal for a stress-relieving bath after a busy day.

Benefits

- **Clears the Mind:** The refreshing aroma of eucalyptus will clear the mental fog and help you attain concentration for relaxation and sleep.
- **Relieves Muscle Tension:** Eucalyptus oil's anti-inflammatory action merges with castor oil's moisturizing action, soothing sore muscles and relaxing body tension.
- **Supports Respiratory Health:** It may further improve respiratory health by clearing the pathways, making breathing more accessible.

How to Make and Use the Tranquil Eucalyptus & Castor Embrace Bath Elixir

Ingredients:

- 1/4 cup of castor oil (cold-pressed and hexane-free)
- 10-15 drops of eucalyptus essential oil
- 1 cup of sea salt or Himalayan pink salt (optional, for additional detoxification)
- A small jar or container for mixing

Instructions:

- **Combine the Ingredients:** In a small jar or other container, mix together the following: castor oil and eucalyptus essential oil. If desired, add sea salt or Himalayan pink salt. Stir until all three components are combined into a uniform mixture.
- **Prepare the Bath:** Fill your tub with hot water. As the tub is filling, add the mixture to the water, gently stirring your hand in the tub to help the oil and salts distribute themselves.

- **Soak and Breathe Deeply:** Fill the tub with warm water, then sink in and take deep breaths of the eucalyptus fragrance, getting a chance to free your mind and set your body at ease. Soak in the bath for 20-30 minutes.
- **Rinse and Revitalize:** Rinse the remaining oil with warm water after soaking. Pat dry your skin and revel in the refreshing, revived sensation.

Usage Tips:

- Use this bath elixir when you need to clear your mind and relieve muscle tension, especially after physical activity or a stressful day.
- Store any leftover mixture in a cool, dark place, and shake well before each use.

Calm Chamomile & Castor Bath Bedtime

Why It Works

Chamomile is a gentle and mild herb that supports relaxation by offering anti-inflammatory and calming properties. It has been used for ages to promote sleep and anxiety reduction, especially in enhancing sleeping conditions. Mixed with castor oil, which moisturizes deep into the skin, it makes for a relaxing environment since one is supposed to go to sleep afterward.

Benefits

- **Promotes Relaxation:** Chamomile's calming nature relaxes the mind and body, helping individuals prepare for sleep.

- **Soothes the Skin:** Chamomile is popularly known for soothing skin and is ideal for persons with sensitive or irritated skin. It combines well with castor oil to moisturize and soothe the skin.
- **Enhances Sleep Quality:** Chamomile baths before sleeping contribute to a decrease in stress and anxiety, which means that sleep will be much deeper and more qualitative.

How to Make and Use the Calm Chamomile & Castor Bath Bedtime

Ingredients:

- 1/4 cup of castor oil (cold-pressed and hexane-free)
- 10-15 drops of chamomile essential oil or 2 chamomile tea bags
- 1 cup of oatmeal (optional, for added skin-soothing benefits)
- A small jar or container for mixing

Instructions:

- **Combine the Ingredients:** Mix the castor oil with the chamomile essential oil in a small jar or container. If using tea bags, steep in a cup of hot water for a few minutes until cool, then add the tea to the bath. Add the oatmeal to a muslin bag or cloth and tie it securely.
- **Prepare the Bath:** Fill your bathtub with warm water. While the tub is filling, pour the oil mixture into the water while gently stirring by hand to help disperse the oil. If you added oatmeal to this batch, then place the muslin bag into the bath.

- **Soak and Unwind:** Soak in the bath for 20-30 minutes, letting the calming smell of chamomile take effect with the moisturizing effects of castor oil on both your body and mind.
- **Rinse and Relax:** Once you are out of your bath, rinse all residual oil from your body using warm water. Pat dry and get ready for a night of sound sleep.

Usage Tips:

- Use this bath blend in the evening to help unwind and promote restful sleep.
- Store any leftover mixture in a cool, dark place, and shake well before each use.

Peaceful Peppermint & Castor Oil Bath Mixture

Why It Works

Peppermint oil rejuvenates the body due to its cooling, refreshing effect. Moreover, it relieves mental fatigue and stress, as well as tension within the muscles. Its refreshing aroma may help untangle a confused mind and foster calmness. The peppermint oil and castor oil mixture for a bath has a soothing effect on the mind and body from probable stress and tension.

Benefits

- **Refreshes the Mind:** Peppermint oil's cooling and invigorating aroma refreshes the mind, eradicating mental fatigue while promoting clarity.
- **Relieves Muscle Tension:** Peppermint oil is also anti-inflammatory, which helps relieve muscle

tension and pain. This makes the bath mixture highly appropriate after a long day or some strenuous activity.

- **Cools and Soothes the Skin:** Peppermint oil cools down the skin, and castor oil hydrates the skin; these two combined to soothe and calm the skin to a refreshed feeling.

How to Make and Use the Peaceful Peppermint & Castor Oil Bath Mixture

Ingredients:

- 1/4 cup of castor oil (cold-pressed and hexane-free)
- 10-15 drops of peppermint essential oil
- 1 cup of baking soda (optional, for added skin softening and detoxifying effects)
- A small jar or container for mixing

Instructions:

- **Combine the Ingredients:** Combine the castor oil and peppermint essential oil in a small jar or container. Add the baking soda, if applicable, and stir to ensure it is well-mixed.
- **Prepare the Bath:** Fill the bathtub with warm water. As it fills, add the mixture, stirring lightly with your hand to help the oil and baking soda disperse.
- **Soak and Refresh:** Fill your tub with water, adding this to the bathwater. Then, soak in it for 20 to 30 minutes to let the refreshing aroma of peppermint and the cooling sensation of the bath mix work its magic on your mind and body.

- **Rinse and Rejuvenate:** After the bath, wash off the remaining oil with warm water. Pat your skin dry and enjoy your refreshed, rejuvenated skin.

Usage Tips:

- Use this bath mixture when you need to refresh your mind and relieve muscle tension, especially after a stressful day.
- Store any leftover mixture in a cool, dark place, and shake well before each use.

Rejuvenating Lemongrass & Castor Oil Blend

Why It Works

Obtained from a type of grass, lemongrass essential oil is widely known for its refreshing, minty citrus aroma. It also relaxes stress and uplifts mood while rejuvenating the mind and body. It has anti-microbial and anti-inflammatory properties that can be used to soothe the skin. Blended with castor oil, lemongrass creates a rejuvenating bath blend that energizes the body while offering deep relaxation in its own way.

Benefits

- **Uplifts the Mood:** Lemongrass essential oil lightens the mood with its grassy and citrus aroma and helps reduce stress, enhancing overall well-being.
- **Rejuvenates the Body:** The refreshing properties of lemongrass oil and the moisturizing effects of castor oil rejuvenate the tired body; hence, it is perfect either to wake up fresh in the morning or as a reliever after a day's work.

- **Soothes the Skin:** Lemongrass oil's anti-inflammatory properties soothe and calm the skin, while castor oil deeply hydrates it.

How to Make and Use the Rejuvenating Lemongrass & Castor Oil Blend

Ingredients:

- 1/4 cup of castor oil (cold-pressed and hexane-free)
- 10-15 drops of lemongrass essential oil
- 1/2 cup of Epsom salts (optional, for added muscle relaxation)
- A small jar or container for mixing

Instructions:

- **Combine the Ingredients:** In a small jar or container, combine the castor oil and lemongrass essential oil. Add Epsom salts if you are using them. Mix until all three ingredients are fully incorporated.
- **Prepare the Bath:** Fill your bathtub with warm water. As the tub fills, pour the mixture into the water, gently stirring with your hand to help the oil and salts distribute throughout the water.
- **Soak and Rejuvenate:** Fill the tub with water and soak in it for 20-30 minutes. As the refreshing aroma of lemongrass fills your senses, let the refreshing action of the bath blend uplift your mood and rejuvenate your body.
- **Rinse and Energize:** After bathing, wash off the excess oil from your body with warm water. Pat your skin dry, and you will feel energized and rejuvenated.

Usage Tips:

- Use this bath blend to start your day with energy and positivity, or in the evening to rejuvenate after a long day.
- Store any leftover mixture in a cool, dark place, and shake well before each use.

These blends introduced into your personal care will effectively manage stress, ensure relaxation, and promote overall well-being. From the Soothing Lavender & Castor Oil Bath Soak, the Tranquil Eucalyptus & Castor Embrace Bath Elixir, the Calm Chamomile & Castor Bath Bedtime, the Peaceful Peppermint & Castor Oil Bath Mixture, down to the Rejuvenating Lemongrass & Castor Oil Blend, each of them has various benefits associated with helping one relax, regain energy, and rejuvenate.

Blending the therapeutic properties of essential oils with the moisturizing and nourishing properties of castor oil, these bath blends create a truly sensual and effective way to relieve stress and promote relaxation. Whether one wishes to bring calmness into the evening hours, alleviate muscle soreness, or enjoy a peaceful moment, they are a perfect natural remedy for all such requests.

Take a moment to enjoy these stress-releasing bath mixtures and the many ways each mixture will help your mind, body, and soul. Welcome the calm of a warm, soothing bath as natural ingredients get to work on making you feel refreshed, relaxed, and ready to take on life once again with renewed vitality and calmness.

Aromatherapy Oils for Anxiety

Anxiety is among the most widespread disorders; it affects millions of people worldwide and mostly manifests itself in the form of feelings of worry, nervousness, or unease. With various treatments, many people seek nature to assist with their anxiety. Aromatherapy, where essential oils are used to help improve conditions in mental and physical well-being, has thus been an effective tool in reducing anxiety and promoting relaxation. These can be utilized in various forms, including bath drops, massage oils, or wellness potions, with the assistance of castor oil, a nourishing carrier oil, to help ease anxiety and restore balance. The following section highlights, among others, five of the best aromatherapy blends: soothing ylang-ylang and castor aromatic oil, zen bergamot and castor oil bath drops, rosemary and Castor balancing bath potion, jasmine and Castor harmonious bath therapy, and frankincense and Castor serene wellness oil.

Easing Ylang Ylang & Castor Aromatic Oil

Why It Works

Ylang-Ylang oil is sweet-scented and floral; its properties are mainly towards promoting relaxation and soothing the nervous system. In such instances, it dispels anxiety and stress, and hence it should be a consideration when the levels of anxiety are high. These become even more effectual when combined with castor oil, which delivers the essential oil deep in the skin while nourishing and moisturizing it.

Benefits

- **Calms the Nervous System:** The sweet fragrance of Ylang Ylang has a soothing effect on the nervous system and pacifies bouts of anxiety that usher in peace.

- **Promotes Emotional Balance:** The floral fragrance of Ylang Ylang uplifts a person's mood and balances their emotions in order to handle stress and anxiety better.
- **Nourishes the Skin:** Ricinoleic acid makes Castor oil rich in moisture content; hence, it hydrates and nourishes skin for smoothness.

How to Make and Use the Easing Ylang Ylang & Castor Aromatic Oil

Ingredients:

- 2 tablespoons of castor oil (cold-pressed and hexane-free)
- 10-15 drops of Ylang Ylang essential oil
- A small glass bottle with a dropper for storage

Instructions:

- **Combine the Ingredients:** Mix these ingredients together in a small glass bottle. Add the castor oil to the Ylang Ylang essential oil in a glass bottle and mix well, shaking to combine the oils.
- **Application:** Place a few drops of the aromatic oil on your pulse points, such as the wrists, temples, and behind the ears. Gently massage the oil into your skin, inhaling the soothing scent of Ylang Ylang.
- **Relax and Breathe:** Take a few deep breaths, letting the calming aroma help you relax and dilute anxiety.

Usage Tips:

- Use this aromatic oil as needed throughout the day to help manage anxiety and stress.
- Store the bottle in a cool, dark place to preserve the potency of the essential oils.

Zen Bergamot & Castor Oil Bath Drops

Why It Works

It is celebrated for its fresh, citrusy scent and for curing anxiety and depression. It uplifts one's mood by decreasing anxiety, sadness, and stress. Bergamot has good blending properties, and taken in combination with the nutty castor oil for a warm bath, bergamot essential oil is a good choice to cleanse and build mental clarity and emotional balance.

Benefits

- **Alleviates Anxiety and Depression:** The uplifting perfume of Bergamot tends to reduce anxious feelings and depression, therefore increasing well-being.
- **Promotes Mental Clarity:** Fresh and citrusy, the subtle perfume of Bergamot opens the mind and diminishes foggy cerebral states, promoting clarity and focused attention.
- **Moisturizes the Skin:** Castor oil is rich in emollient properties, thus helping with skin moisturizing and soothing.

How to Make and Use the Zen Bergamot & Castor Oil Bath Drops

Ingredients:

- 2 tablespoons of castor oil (cold-pressed and hexane-free)
- 10-15 drops of Bergamot essential oil
- A small glass bottle with a dropper for storage

Instructions:

- **Combine the Ingredients:** Add the bergamot essential oil to castor oil in a small glass bottle. Shake well to mix the oils properly.
- **Prepare the Bath:** Fill your tub with warm water. Add 5-10 drops of Zen Bergamot & Castor Oil Bath Drops to the water, gently stirring with your hand to help disperse the oil.
- **Soak and Relax:** Soak the body in the tub for 20-30 minutes while the uplifting Bergamot fragrance soothes the mind and loosens up anxiety.

Usage Tips:

- Use these bath drops in the evening to unwind after a stressful day or whenever you need a mood boost.
- Store the bottle in a cool, dark place to preserve the potency of the essential oils.

Balancing Rosemary & Castor Bath Potion

Why It Works

Rosemary essential oil awakens the mind and increases alertness. It also has grounding properties and is capable of balancing emotional responses to prevent anxiety. Therefore, it is great for people who feel swamped or stressed. Castor oil, on the other hand, feeds and soothes the skin. Therefore, this bath potion with castor oil will help restore your emotional balance and promote calmness.

Benefits

- **Promotes Mental Clarity:** It relieves mental fogginess through its stimulating effect by promoting clarity and concentration, hence acting as an enormous reliever in stressful, anxious states of mind and body.
- **Balances Emotions:** The aroma of rosemary is centring. Once the feelings become balanced, the feeling of being overwhelmed decreases, hence decreasing stress.
- **Nourishes the Skin:** Castor oil's moisturizing effects help hydrate and nourish the skin, leaving it soft and supple.

How to Make and Use the Balancing Rosemary & Castor Bath Potion

Ingredients:

- 2 tablespoons of castor oil (cold-pressed and hexane-free)
- 10-15 drops of Rosemary essential oil
- 1 cup of Epsom salts (optional, for additional muscle relaxation)
- A small jar or container for mixing

Instructions:

- **Combine the Ingredients:** In a small jar or container, combine the castor oil with the Rosemary essential oil. Add the Epsom salts to that mixture if using. Stir well to make sure all the ingredients are well combined.
- **Prepare the Bath:** Fill your bathtub with warm water. While the tub is filling up, pour the mixture into the water, gently stirring with your hand to help the oil and salts disperse.
- **Soak and Balance:** Sit in the bath for 20-30 minutes, relaxing while Rosemary takes its grounding action and castor oil moisturizes to balance and soothe.

Usage Tips:

- Use this bath potion when you need to clear your mind and restore emotional balance, especially after a stressful day.
- Store any leftover mixture in a cool, dark place, and shake well before each use.

Harmonious Jasmine & Castor Bath Therapy

Why It Works

Jasmine essential oil has been valued for its sweet, floral fragrance and its ability to uplift mood and reduce anxiety. Due to its calming effect on the nervous system, it works well for those who are under tremendous stress and suffer from emotional exhaustion. Coupled with castor oil, jasmine provides this indulging bath therapy that facilitates relaxation and emotional harmony.

Benefits

- **Uplifts the Mood:** Jasmine's lively smell tends to lessen anxiety, elevating an individual's mood and making him joyful and well.
- **Promotes Emotional Harmony:** Jasmine has soothing properties for the emotions. This keeps stress and emotional exhaustion at bay because of its balancing nature on the emotional level.
- Moisturizes and Nourishes the Skin: Castor oil is rich in moisturizing and nourishment capabilities that keep the skin hydrated, leaving it soft and smooth with a radiating glow.

How to Make and Use the Harmonious Jasmine & Castor Bath Therapy

Ingredients:

- 2 tablespoons of castor oil (cold-pressed and hexane-free)
- 10-15 drops of Jasmine essential oil
- 1 cup of coconut milk (optional, for added skin nourishment)
- A small jar or container for mixing

Instructions:

- Combine the Ingredients: Combine castor oil with Jasmine essential oil in a small jar or container. If desired, stir in the coconut milk. Make sure the ingredients are well incorporated.
- Prepare the Bath: Fill your bathtub with warm water. As it fills, pour the mixture into the water, allowing your hand to stir the mixture; this will help the dispersion of oil and milk.

- Soak and Harmonize: Soak in this bath for 20-30 minutes while the sweet fragrance of Jasmine uplifts and castor oil moisturizes to balance your emotions.

Usage Tips:

- Use this bath therapy when you need to uplift your spirits and restore emotional balance.
- Store any leftover mixture in a cool, dark place, and shake well before each use.

Serene Frankincense & Castor Wellness Oil

Why It Works

Frankincense essential oil has a very grounding effect; its calming effects are highly recommended. For ages, it has been used during spiritual and religious activities to provide a feeling of peace and tranquillity. It is effective at reducing anxiety and promoting a sense of well-being. This wellness oil, therefore, becomes a powerful tool in calming both mind and body in combination with castor oil, making it an excellent choice in the management of anxiety.

Benefits

- **Promotes Inner Peace:** Frankincense has a grounding aroma that helps to relax the head and keep the soul tranquil.
- **Reduces Anxiety:** Frankincense makes an individual calm from stress factors responsible for anxiety, hence promoting well-being.
- **Nourishes the Skin:** Castor oil has moisturizing effects; it nourishes and keeps the skin fresh and hydrated, thus leaving the skin soft and smooth.

How to Make and Use the Serene Frankincense & Castor Wellness Oil

Ingredients:

- 2 tablespoons of castor oil (cold-pressed and hexane-free)
- 10-15 drops of Frankincense essential oil
- A small glass bottle with a dropper for storage

Instructions:

- **Combine the Ingredients:** In a small glass bottle, combine castor oil with Frankincense essential oil. Shake well to combine the oils.
- **Application:** Apply a few drops of this wellness oil to the pulse points of your wrists, temples, and behind your ears. Lightly massage the oil into your skin, inhaling the grounding scent of Frankincense.
- **Relax and Breathe:** Take a few deep breaths, allowing the calming aroma to help reduce anxiety and promote a sense of inner peace.

Usage Tips:

- Use this wellness oil as needed throughout the day to help manage anxiety and promote a sense of well-being.
- Store the bottle in a cool, dark place to preserve the potency of the essential oils.

Aromatherapy is one of the natural, effective means to handle anxiety and promote relaxation. The recipes of aromatherapy blends that follow-Easing Ylang Ylang & Castor Aromatic Oil, Zen Bergamot & Castor Oil Bath Drops, Balancing Rosemary & Castor Bath Potion,

Harmonious Jasmine & Castor Bath Therapy, and Serene Frankincense & Castor Wellness Oil-use the holistic power of essential oils in combination with the nourishing properties of castor oil to create holistic approaches toward easing anxiety and restoring emotional balance.

These can be included in stress management; anxiety will be reduced while peace with one's inner self will be heightened. You can apply the oils to your body, add them to your bath, or exercise meditation. These blends have a natural way of improving mental and emotional health. Allow yourself to let go and rise above with these aromatherapy oils, embracing the next step in the process of keeping anxiety at bay and enhancing overall wellness.

Castor Oil for Babies & Children

Among the most critical concerns of a parent is caring for sensitive skin in babies and children, and many are eager to seek natural, mild treatments that are free of irritants and other chemical additives. Castor oil is rich, moisturizing, and anti-inflammatory, making it an excellent choice for treating various problems with infants and young children's skin. This versatile oil is non-irritating, effective, and can be used in myriad formulations to combat common issues like diaper rash, cradle cap, and dry skin. In the next section, we shall look at the application of castor oil in baby care, from therapeutic applications for diaper rash and cradle caps to mild massage oil.

Oil for Babies

Why It Works

Castor oil is light nat,ural, and harmless to a baby's delicate skin. Its high content of fatty acids, primarily ricinoleic acid, deeply nourishes the skin to protect it from dryness and irritation. Castor oil also possesses antibacterial and anti-inflammatory qualities, thus being well-suited for preventing and treating minor skin problems in infants.

Benefits

- **Deep Moisturization:** Castor oil locks a protective layer in the skin, retaining moisture to prevent dryness.
- **Soothes Irritation:** Its anti-inflammatory properties soothe irritated skin and are excellent for minor rashes or dry patches.
- **Safe for Sensitive Skin:** When properly diluted, castor oil is gentle on even the most sensitive skin of newborns and infants.

How to Use

- **Dilution:** Dilute it with one part castor oil to two parts of lighter carrier oil, such as coconut, almond, or olive oil.
- **Application:** Gently apply the diluted oil to the baby's skin after bath time, particularly to drier or irritated areas. This might also be used more generally as a moisturizer to keep the baby's skin smooth.

Diaper Rash Treatment

Why It Works

Diaper rash is an ordinary condition a baby faces, which usually arises from a highly wet diaper left for a while, rubbing, or allergic sensitivity to the material of the diapers. Castor oil offers soothing and moisturizing action; hence, it forms an excellent base for treating diaper rash. Its thick consistency creates a barrier on the skin that protects it from further irritation; the anti-inflammatory action lessens the redness and discomfort.

Benefits

- **Protects and Heals:** Castor oil protects the baby's skin, allowing it to heal and preventing further irritation.
- **Reduces Inflammation:** Its natural anti-inflammatory properties help soothe redness and discomfort associated with diaper rash.
- **Prevents Future Rashes:** Regularly moisturizing and protecting the baby's skin helps prevent diaper rash.

How to Use

- **Application:** Clean and dry the baby's diaper area. Apply a thin layer of castor oil directly to the affected area after each diaper change to provide relief and keep the skin soothed and protected.

Soothing Diaper Rash Balm

Why It Works

Castor oil is an extra-soothing balm for diaper rash that adds extra protection and heals tender areas of the diaper. Mixed with other natural protective ingredients such as beeswax and shea butter, it will create a balm that not only treats diaper rash but also aids in its prevention due to its moisture barrier, thus helping deliver great nourishment to the skin.

Benefits

- **Creates a Protective Barrier:** A thick barrier covering the skin, a mix of castor oil, shea butter, and beeswax protects the skin from moisture and friction.
- **Deeply Moisturizes:** It deeply moisturizes the rich formula that keeps the baby's skin hydrated, preventing dryness that could lead to skin irritation.
- **Soothes and Heals:** Castor oil's anti-inflammatory properties combine with the nourishing effects of shea butter to heal and soothe diaper rash quickly.

How to Make and Use

Ingredients:

- 2 tablespoons of castor oil
- 2 tablespoons of shea butter
- 1 tablespoon of beeswax pellets

Instructions:

- Melt the shea butter and beeswax in a double boiler.
- Remove from heat and stir in the castor oil until well combined.

- Allow the mixture to cool and solidify in a clean container.
- Apply the balm to the baby's clean, dry diaper area as needed, particularly at bedtime to provide overnight protection.

Anti-Inflammatory Diaper Cream

Why It Works

Castor oil-based anti-inflammatory diaper cream may be very helpful to newborn babies with sensitive skin or suffering from recurrent diaper rash. When calming calendula and chamomile extracts are combined with the inherent anti-inflammatory action of castor oil, it forms a light lotion that reduces redness, inflammation, and swelling.

Benefits

- **Reduces Redness and Swelling:** Calendula, chamomile, and castor oil together help reduce inflammation caused by diaper rash.
- **Gentle on Sensitive Skin:** This cream is mild enough for daily use on even the most sensitive skin.
- **Provides Long-Lasting Moisture:** Castor oil's thick texture keeps skin nourished and protected between diaper changes.

How to Make and Use

Ingredients:

- 2 tablespoons of castor oil
- 1 tablespoon of calendula oil

- 1 tablespoon of chamomile oil
- 1/4 cup of zinc oxide (for added protection)

Instructions:

- In a clean bowl, mix the castor oil with calendula and chamomile oils.
- Gradually stir in the zinc oxide until a smooth cream forms.
- Store in an airtight container.
- Apply to the baby's diaper area during each diaper change to reduce inflammation and protect the skin.

Nourishing Diaper Ointment

Why It Works

Adding castor oil to a rich, emollient ointment on the diaper area helps prevent and heal diaper rash. It also helps smooth and moisturize the baby's skin. Vitamin E oil adds to the ointment's ability to shield and restore sensitive skin.

Benefits

- **Rich Moisturization:** Castor oil's thick consistency locks in moisture, preventing wetness and irritation to the baby's skin.
- **Heals and Protects:** Vitamin E oil adds an extra layer of protection and quickens the healing of broken skin.
- **Prevents Diaper Rash:** Regular application of this ointment prevents diaper rash, as it maintains good barriers that keep moisture from the skin.

How to Make and Use

Ingredients:

- 2 tablespoons of castor oil
- 1 tablespoon of coconut oil
- 1 teaspoon of vitamin E oil

Instructions:

- Combine all ingredients in a clean container and stir well.
- Apply the ointment to the baby's diaper area after each diaper change to keep the skin nourished and protected.

Gentle Diaper Rash Spray

Why It Works

The castor oil base is gentle enough to treat and prevent diaper rash in the spray. This format is easy and convenient for on-the-go application because it allows an easy application onto the skin without having to rub the skin, which may be tender during the rash.

Benefits

- **Easy Application:** The spray format reduces the need for direct skin contact, which is easily irritated; this makes it simpler and less frustrating when it comes to quick, easy application.
- **Soothes and Protects:** Castor oil soothes diaper rash and forms a thin, impermeable barrier on the skin.
- **Hydrates:** The spray helps to hydrate the skin, reducing the chance of another rash appearing.

How to Make and Use

Ingredients:

- 2 tablespoons of castor oil
- 2 tablespoons of distilled water
- 1 tablespoon of witch hazel (optional, for extra soothing)

Instructions:

- Mix all ingredients in a clean spray bottle and shake well before each use.
- Spray directly onto the baby's diaper area during each diaper change.
- Allow to air dry before putting on a clean diaper.

Herbal Diaper Rash Salve

Why It Works

An herbal diaper rash salve prepared with castor oil and the natural art of infusion with soothing herbs such as calendula, chamomile, and lavender provides an absolutely gentle, natural treatment for diaper rash. The herbs add to the extra anti-inflammatory and healing properties, which make this salve very effective for severe or stubborn diaper rash.

Benefits

- **Herbal Healing:** Castor oil combined with healing herbs helps quickly pacify diaper rash.
- **Moisturizes and Protects:** Castor oil protects the skin with its moisturizing feature, while herbal infusion does extra work of protecting against irritation.

- **Gentle on Skin:** The salve is light enough for even the most sensitive skin and soothes without irritation.

How to Make and Use

Ingredients:

- 2 tablespoons of castor oil
- 1 tablespoon of calendula oil
- 1 tablespoon of chamomile oil
- 10 drops of lavender essential oil

Instructions:

- Combine all ingredients in a clean container and stir well.
- Apply the salve to the baby's diaper area after each diaper change to soothe and heal the skin.

Natural Remedies for Cradle Cap

Cradle cap in babies is generally characterized by scaly and dry patches on the Scalp. It isn't dangerous, yet it doesn't look lovely and may be very discomforting for the baby. Castor oil, being moisturizing and anti-inflammatory in nature, helps soften the scales, thus helping them easily remove while nourishing the Scalp.

Why It Works

- **Moisturizes the Scalp:** Castor oil's richness emolliates the dry, scaly patches associated with the cradle cap.
- **Promotes Healing:** Anti-inflammatory properties soothe the scalp and promote healing.

- **Gentle and Safe:** Castor oil is mild enough for even the most sensitive baby scalps. Without causing any irritation, it effectively treats the disorder.

Cradle Cap Treatment Oil

Why It Works

The scaling on the scalp might get loosened with a cradle cap treatment oil prepared with castor oil, which could be easily brushed off. This treatment oil can be further enriched by incorporating soothing oils like jojoba or almond oil to enhance nourishment.

Benefits

- Softens Scales: The castor oil helps the thick, scaly patches soften so that they are easier to remove.
- Nourishes the Scalp: This oil deeply penetrates the scalp, letting moisture in to create a healthy environment.
- Gentle on Baby's Skin: This treatment is very gentle and safe, designed for the tender skin of a baby.

How to Make and Use

Ingredients:

- 2 tablespoons of castor oil
- 1 tablespoon of jojoba oil (optional)
- 1 tablespoon of almond oil (optional)

Instructions:

- Mix the oils together in a clean container.

- Apply a small amount of the oil to the affected areas of the baby's scalp, massaging gently.
- Leave on for 15-20 minutes to allow the oil to soften the scales.
- Gently brush the scalp with a soft-bristled brush to remove the softened scales.
- Wash the baby's hair with a gentle baby shampoo to remove any excess oil.

Gentle Cradle Cap Scrub

Why It Works

A light cradle cap scrub made with castor oil and a gentle exfoliant, such as ground oatmeal or baking soda, helps to exfoliate the scalp and remove the flakes with scales that come with cradle cap.

Benefits

- **Exfoliates Gently:** The mild exfoliating agent helps remove the scales without further irritating the sensitive scalp of the baby.
- **Moisturizes and Protects:** Castor oil deeply moisturizes and protects the scalp.
- **Promotes Healing:** The scrub allows the scalp to be clean and healthy, thus giving an avenue for the cradle cap to heal faster.

How to Make and Use

Ingredients:

- 2 tablespoons of castor oil
- 1 tablespoon of ground oatmeal or baking soda

Instructions:

- Mix the castor oil with the ground oatmeal or baking soda to form a paste.
- Apply the scrub to the affected areas of the scalp, gently massaging in circular motions.
- Leave on for 5-10 minutes to allow the oil to moisturize and the exfoliant to work.
- Rinse off with warm water and gently wash the baby's hair with a mild shampoo.

Herbal Infused Cradle Cap Oil

Why It Works

Such a cradle cap herbal-infused oil, which includes castor oil and soothing herbs such as calendula and chamomile, has become a really nourishing and soothing treatment for the baby's scalp.

Benefits

- **Herbal Healing:** The healing action of the infusion works to soothe and heal the scalp, reducing irritation while keeping the skin healthy.
- **Softens and Moisturizes:** Castor oil deeply moisturizes the scalp while softening the scales for easy removal.
- **Safe and Gentle:** This treatment is soft enough to be used on a baby's delicate scalp.

How to Make and Use

Ingredients:

- 2 tablespoons of castor oil
- 1 tablespoon of calendula oil

- 1 tablespoon of chamomile oil

Instructions:

- Combine all ingredients in a clean container and stir well.
- Apply the oil to the affected areas of the scalp, massaging gently.
- Leave on for 15-20 minutes to allow the oil to soften the scales.
- Gently brush the scalp with a soft-bristled brush to remove the softened scales.
- Wash the baby's hair with a gentle baby shampoo to remove any excess oil.

Moisturizing Cradle Cap Lotion

Why It Works

This castor oil-based cradle cap lotion will help keep the dry, flaky scalp of a baby moisturized and soothed with the addition of aloe vera and shea butter.

Benefits

- **Deep Hydration:** The combination of castor oil, aloe vera, and shea butter deeply hydrates the skin to help smoothen and remove the scales.
- **Soothes Irritation:** Aloe vera helps to soothe irritation and reduces any form of inflammation, hence promoting the healing process on the scalp.
- **Nourishes the Scalp:** he ingredients Shea butter and castor oil will nourish the scalp, protect it, and thus avoid further dryness and irritation.

How to Make and Use

Ingredients:

- 2 tablespoons of castor oil
- 2 tablespoons of aloe vera gel
- 1 tablespoon of shea butter

Instructions:

- Melt the shea butter in a double boiler.
- Remove from heat and stir in the castor oil and aloe vera gel until well combined.
- Allow the mixture to cool and solidify in a clean container.
- Apply the lotion to the baby's scalp, gently massaging it in.
- Leave on for 15-20 minutes, then rinse off with warm water and wash the baby's hair with a mild shampoo.

Aloe & Castor Cradle Cap Gel

Why It Works

A cradle cap gel made with castor oil and aloe vera provides a soothing and moisturizing treatment that is easy to apply and absorbs quickly into the scalp.

Benefits

- **Soothes and Moisturizes:** Aloe vera provides soothing hydration, while castor oil helps to lock in moisture and protect the scalp.
- **Softens Scales:** The gel consistency makes it easy to apply and helps to soften the dry, flaky patches associated with cradle cap.

- **Gentle Formula:** This gel is gentle enough for daily use and is safe for a baby's delicate scalp.

How to Make and Use

Ingredients:

- 2 tablespoons of castor oil
- 2 tablespoons of aloe vera gel

Instructions:

- Mix the castor oil and aloe vera gel together in a clean container.
- Apply a small amount of the gel to the affected areas of the scalp, massaging gently.
- Leave on for 15-20 minutes, then gently rinse off with warm water.
- Wash the baby's hair with a mild shampoo to remove any remaining gel.

Gentle Cradle Cap Treatment

Why It Works

A gentle cradle cap treatment made with castor oil and chamomile provides a soothing and effective remedy for babies suffering from cradle cap. Chamomile's anti-inflammatory properties help to reduce irritation, while castor oil softens and moisturizes the scalp.

Benefits

- **Reduces Inflammation:** Chamomile helps to reduce inflammation and soothe the scalp, making it easier to remove the scales.

- **Moisturizes and Protects:** Castor oil keeps the scalp moisturized, preventing further dryness and irritation.
- **Safe for Sensitive Skin:** This treatment is gentle and safe for use on a baby's delicate scalp.

How to Make and Use

Ingredients:

- 2 tablespoons of castor oil
- 1 tablespoon of chamomile oil

Instructions:

- Combine the castor oil and chamomile oil in a clean container.
- Apply a small amount of the oil to the affected areas of the scalp, massaging gently.
- Leave on for 15-20 minutes, then rinse off with warm water.
- Gently brush the scalp with a soft-bristled brush to remove the softened scales.

Gentle Massage Oils for Babies

Baby massage is a wonderful way to bond with your infant while promoting relaxation, better sleep, and healthy skin. Massage oils made with castor oil can enhance the benefits of massage by providing deep hydration and nourishment to the baby's skin. Below are some gentle and calming massage oil blends specifically designed for babies.

Calming Baby Massage Oil

Why It Works

A calming baby massage oil made with castor oil and lavender essential oil provides a soothing and relaxing experience for both baby and parent. Lavender's calming scent helps to relax the baby and prepare them for sleep, while castor oil nourishes and protects the skin.

Benefits

- **Promotes Relaxation:** Lavender's calming properties help to soothe the baby, making it easier for them to relax and fall asleep.
- **Nourishes the Skin:** Castor oil provides deep hydration and nourishment, keeping the baby's skin soft and smooth.
- **Gentle and Safe:** This massage oil is gentle enough for daily use and is safe for even the most sensitive skin.

How to Make and Use

Ingredients:

- 2 tablespoons of castor oil
- 5 drops of lavender essential oil

Instructions:

- Combine the castor oil and lavender essential oil in a clean container.
- Warm the oil slightly by placing the container in a bowl of warm water.
- Apply the oil to your hands and gently massage the baby's skin, focusing on the arms, legs, and back.

- Use gentle, circular motions to help the baby relax and enjoy the massage.

Nourishing Baby Massage Oil

Why It Works

A nourishing baby massage oil made with castor oil and almond oil provides intense moisture and nourishment to the baby's skin. Almond oil is rich in vitamins A and E, which help to keep the skin healthy and protected.

Benefits

- **Deeply Moisturizes:** The combination of castor oil and almond oil provides deep hydration, making this oil perfect for babies with dry or sensitive skin.
- **Nourishes and Protects:** The vitamins in almond oil help to nourish and protect the baby's skin, keeping it healthy and soft.
- **Gentle Formula:** This massage oil is gentle enough for daily use and is safe for all skin types.

How to Make and Use

Ingredients:

- 2 tablespoons of castor oil
- 2 tablespoons of almond oil

Instructions:

- Combine the castor oil and almond oil in a clean container.
- Warm the oil slightly by placing the container in a bowl of warm water.

- Apply the oil to your hands and gently massage the baby's skin, focusing on dry or sensitive areas.
- Use gentle, circular motions to help the baby relax and enjoy the massage.

Soothing Lavender Baby Oil

Why It Works

Soothing lavender baby oil made with castor oil and lavender essential oil offers calming benefits that help reduce stress and promote sleep in babies. This blend is ideal for use after bath time or before bedtime to help prepare the baby for a restful night.

Benefits

- **Calms and Soothes:** Lavender essential oil helps to calm the baby and reduce anxiety, making it easier for them to sleep.
- **Moisturizes the Skin:** Castor oil provides deep hydration, keeping the baby's skin soft and smooth.
- **Gentle and Safe:** This baby oil is formulated to be gentle on sensitive skin, making it safe for daily use.

How to Make and Use

Ingredients:

- 2 tablespoons of castor oil
- 5 drops of lavender essential oil

Instructions:

- Mix the castor oil with the lavender essential oil in a clean container.

- Warm the oil slightly by placing the container in a bowl of warm water.
- Apply the oil to the baby's skin after bath time or before bedtime, using gentle massage strokes to help them relax.

Hydrating Baby Body Oil

Why It Works

A hydrating baby body oil made with castor oil and coconut oil provides intense moisture and protection for the baby's delicate skin. Coconut oil is rich in fatty acids that help to lock in moisture and protect the skin from dryness and irritation.

Benefits

- **Intense Hydration:** The combination of castor oil and coconut oil provides deep hydration, making this body oil perfect for babies with dry or sensitive skin.
- **Protects the Skin:** Coconut oil helps to create a protective barrier on the skin, preventing moisture loss and keeping the skin soft and smooth.
- **Gentle Formula:** This body oil is gentle enough for daily use and is safe for all skin types.

How to Make and Use

Ingredients:

- 2 tablespoons of castor oil
- 2 tablespoons of coconut oil

Instructions:

- Combine the castor oil and coconut oil in a clean container.

- Warm the oil slightly by placing the container in a bowl of warm water.
- Apply the oil to the baby's skin after bath time, using gentle massage strokes to help them relax and enjoy the moisturizing benefits.

Bedtime Bliss Massage Oil

Why It Works

A bedtime bliss massage oil made with castor oil and a blend of calming essential oils like lavender, chamomile, and sandalwood helps to prepare the baby for a restful night's sleep. This blend creates a soothing, peaceful environment that promotes relaxation and reduces bedtime anxiety.

Benefits

- **Promotes Relaxation:** The calming blend of essential oils helps to relax the baby and prepare them for sleep.
- **Nourishes and Protects:** Castor oil provides deep hydration and protection, keeping the baby's skin soft and smooth.
- **Gentle and Safe:** This massage oil is gentle enough for daily use and is safe for even the most sensitive skin.

How to Make and Use

Ingredients:

- 2 tablespoons of castor oil
- 3 drops of lavender essential oil
- 3 drops of chamomile essential oil
- 2 drops of sandalwood essential oil

Instructions:

- Mix the castor oil with the essential oils in a clean container.
- Warm the oil slightly by placing the container in a bowl of warm water.
- Apply the oil to the baby's skin before bedtime, using gentle massage strokes to help them relax and prepare for sleep.

Castor oil is a versatile and natural solution for caring for babies and children's delicate skin. Whether you're treating diaper rash, cradle cap, or simply looking to nourish and protect your baby's skin, the above formulations offer safe, effective, and gentle ways to incorporate castor oil into your baby's skincare routine. From soothing diaper rash treatments to gentle massage oils that promote relaxation and better sleep, castor oil can play a vital role in keeping your baby's skin healthy, hydrated, and protected.

Chapter 6:
Science-Validated Healing: Why Castor Oil Works at the Cellular Level

Castor oil has been taken both internally and externally for thousands of years as an absolutely natural remedy for arthritis and skin problems. Castor oil serves multiple purposes for both beauty and health; however, what really sets this oil apart is the science supporting its effectiveness. This chapter will elaborate on the chemistry of castor oil, scientific research supporting health benefits, and dispel some of the more common myths and misunderstandings regarding its application. This understanding of the science of castor oil will finally allow you to confidently incorporate it into your holistic program in the full knowledge that the benefits are not only time-tested but proven.

Why is castor oil so effective? What is its chemistry?

Castor oil differs from other plant oils due to its peculiar chemical composition, actually the root of all its might. The oil contains roughly 90% of the fatty acid ricinoleic acid, which actually is responsible for most of its incredible properties. Most of its medicinal properties and even its viscous nature can be attributed to this acid.

The rare fatty acid ricinoleic acid has impressive anti-inflammatory, antibacterial, and moisturizing effects. This deeply infiltrates skin and tissues, allowing for better hydration, anti-inflammation, and anti-infection properties in the skin. Castor oil contains ricinoleic acid, which allows deep permeability into the skin compared to any other oil type, thus keeping the skin hydrated and healing for a longer period of time.

Anti-Inflammatory Action: Anti-inflammatory in nature, ricinoleic acid blocks the production of pro-inflammatory chemicals, thus helping reduce pain, inflammation, and swelling. It is very useful in cases of arthritis, joint pain, and skin irritation. Antimicrobial Action: Basically, Ricinoleic acid is very efficient in treating infections, acne, and other skin disorders because of the fact that besides anti-inflammatory action, this acid has the ability to fight bacteria, fungi, and viruses.

Other Triglycerides and Fatty Acids: Apart from ricinoleic acid, there are other triglycerides and fatty acids in castor oil that contribute to its effectiveness. The fatty acids present in this substance are capable of retaining water; hence, castor oil is an effective home remedy for dry skin, scalp, and hair.

Deep moisturizing: castor oil triglycerides act like a barrier, imparting their ability to the skin to lock moisture and accelerate the healing process. This is why castor oil is so effective in treatments such as psoriasis, eczema, and very dry skin.

High viscosity: Castor oil is viscous, which allows it to stay on the skin and hair for longer periods of time than many other oils, giving nutrients full action to impart long-lasting healing. Due to its viscous nature, it is typically used in hair masks and skin treatments as a carrier oil for other medicinal substances.

The benefits of using castor oil are many, but understanding just why it is so beneficial requires taking a closer look at the chemistry behind it. The makeup of this oil allows it to nourish and heal cells from the inside out, as well as work as a topical treatment, achieving goals that other oils and treatments simply cannot.

Castor Oil Research: Evidence of Skin, Hair, and Joint Benefits

The many health benefits associated with castor oil are now emerging through modern research, though traditional medicine has for years used it. Generations have passed down that castor oil is one of the most strong and helpful organic treatments for a wide range of health problems; several scientific investigations have confirmed this.

Skin Health and Moisturizing: Castor oil raises in hydration and flexibility of the skin up to the extreme, as shown in the study published in the Journal of Cosmetic Science. Therefore, it works magic on stretch marks, wrinkles, or dry skin because the emollient qualities of the oil keep moisture within the skin.

Study Outcome: Topical application of castor oil reduced fine lines and wrinkles, hence generally improving skin moisture. This justifies its application as a natural moisturizer and anti-aging agent.

Hair Growth and Strengthening: It has been proved through scientific research that castor oil encourages hair growth. A study done on the use of ricinoleic acid for hair growth had remarkably increased hair density of participants, and reduced hair loss with castor oil treatment.

It is said to be due to its ability to feed hair follicles and boost the flow of blood to the scalp.

Results of the Study: The regular application of castor oil to the scalp reduced and improved hair thickness and hair loss, respectively. It was further found to stimulate hair growth in areas suffering from alopecia (hair loss).

Joint Health and Pain Relief: Much research has taken place on the anti-inflammatory properties of castor oil and how this will then impact pain, both in muscles and joints. In fact, one study published in the Journal of Medicinal Plants Research showed that applying topical applications of castor oil to arthritis patients had significant reductions in the patient's symptoms of pain and inflammation.

It was established that topical application of castor oil pack to the joints reduces stiffness and discomfort in the results shown in this present study. This, therefore, justifies the use of castor oil as a home remedy treatment for inflammatory disorders such as arthritis.

These scientific investigations confirm the anecdotal benefits long reported by castor oil consumers. Castor oil is a nontoxic natural medication, clinically proven to moisturize the skin, encourage hair growth, and reduce inflammation.

Myths Explosion: Separating Fact from Fiction

Castor oil is endowed with many health benefits, but despite everything, several misconceptions and false beliefs are associated with the oil. Some notions seem to prevail with time and have managed to instill doubts in the minds of potential users. We will now discuss a few of the most prevalent myths in detail and, with the help of scientific data, try to clear the doubts.

Myth 1: Castor Oil is a Cause of Hair Loss: This is one of the biggest myths associated with castor oil and is utterly false. In fact, studies have proved that castor oil enhances hair growth and is particularly helpful for those suffering from baldness or who have thinned their hair. It works perfectly as a hair treatment for regrowth instead of hair loss because it increases blood circulation to the scalp and nurtures hair follicles.

Myth 2: Castor oil is unsafe to use regularly

Factual statement: Castor oil is commonly regarded as safe both for oral intake and topical use on a regular basis. As with any alternative medicine, it is advisable that it be used sparingly. Topical applications of castor oil should not pose any problems, particularly if the type one uses is of good quality, cold-pressed, and hexane-free. When taken internally, it may be safe to act as a laxative, but too much intake may result in addiction or dehydration. Taken as directed, castor oil is safe for use over a period of time.

Myth 3: Castor Oil Is Only Useful to Beautify Fact: While castor oil is indeed famous for nourishing the skin and promoting hair growth, its medical properties are far more extensive than just cosmetic purposes. It has been proved that castor oil relieves joint pain and inflammation; it also improves immunological functioning by stimulating lymphatic flow. With all these uses, it becomes quite handy for health and beauty.

Myth 4: All castor oil products are the same.

Fact: The quality of castor oil may vary dramatically depending on how it is treated. The best-quality oils are cold-pressed, organic, and free from hexane, as they preserve much of the nutritious value inside the oil. Lower qualities of castor oil will not provide as many benefits, and may even cause skin irritation, especially if heated or chemically treated. To get the best results, a high-quality product should be used.

The removal of these rumors makes castor oil more understandable and readers can confidently use it for various health and cosmetic applications.

In Chapter 6, we looked at the scientific basis of the popular application of castor oil as a natural remedy. Indeed, its anti-inflammatory, moisturizing, and restorative properties are second to none and find their source in the peculiar chemistry of the castor oil, especially in the high content of ricinoleic acid within. Various scientific research has shown that castor oil is efficient for hair growth, skin hydration, and even joint pain treatment. Moreover, the clarification of standard misunderstanding about castor oil was a big finding that proved the efficiency and safety of such oil and helped readers to trust in using it on a daily basis.

This chapter makes it very clear that castor oil is indeed a powerful tool for health and beauty, not only for being an effective traditional remedy but also because its efficacy has been validated by modern studies. The therapeutic properties of castor oil act at the cellular level, a guarantee of evident and long-lasting results as far as hair growth, inflammation reduction, or skin elasticity improvement is concerned.

Part 3: 250+ Castor Oil Uses and Remedies

Chapter 7:
Everyday Applications for Skin and Hair

50+ Skin Care Recipes for Radiant, Healthy Skin

Castor oil is probably one of the most effective and multi-purpose natural ingredients in skin care products for all skin types. Its moisturizing, anti-inflammatory, and antibacterial actions will render it perfect for a different array of homemade skincare treatments that may be able to address anything from irritation and aging to dryness and acne. In this section, we add more than 50 castor oil-infused skin care recipes that will help you achieve glowing, healthy skin.

Moisturizing Face Cream for Dry Skin

Ingredients:

- 2 tablespoons of castor oil
- 2 tablespoons of shea butter
- 1 tablespoon of coconut oil
- A few drops of lavender essential oil

Instructions:

- Melt the shea butter and coconut oil in a double boiler.
- Stir in the castor oil and lavender essential oil.
- Allow the mixture to cool and solidify, then whip it into a cream.
- Apply to clean skin, focusing on dry areas.

Anti-Aging Night Serum

Ingredients:

- 1 tablespoon of castor oil
- 1 tablespoon of rosehip oil
- 5 drops of frankincense essential oil

Instructions:

- Mix all the ingredients in a small glass bottle.
- Apply a few drops to your face and neck before bed, focusing on areas prone to wrinkles and fine lines.

Deep Cleansing Oil for Acne-Prone Skin

Ingredients:

- 1 tablespoon of castor oil
- 2 tablespoons of jojoba oil
- 5 drops of tea tree essential oil

Instructions:

- Combine the oils in a small bottle.
- Massage the oil blend into your skin for several minutes to dissolve impurities and makeup.
- Wipe away with a warm, damp cloth.

Brightening Face Mask

Ingredients:

- 1 tablespoon of castor oil
- 1 tablespoon of honey
- 1 tablespoon of lemon juice

Instructions:

- Mix the ingredients into a smooth paste.
- Apply the mask to your face, avoiding the eye area.
- Leave on for 15-20 minutes, then rinse off with warm water.

Gentle Exfoliating Scrub

Ingredients:

- 2 tablespoons of castor oil
- 1 tablespoon of finely ground oats
- 1 tablespoon of honey

Instructions:

- Combine the ingredients in a bowl.
- Massage the scrub onto damp skin in gentle, circular motions.
- Rinse off with warm water and pat dry.

Hydrating Eye Cream

Ingredients:

- 1 tablespoon of castor oil
- 1 tablespoon of almond oil
- 1 tablespoon of aloe vera gel

Instructions:

- Mix all ingredients in a small jar.
- Apply a small amount around the eyes before bed to reduce puffiness and fine lines.

Soothing Body Lotion

Ingredients:

- 2 tablespoons of castor oil
- 2 tablespoons of cocoa butter
- 1 tablespoon of almond oil
- A few drops of chamomile essential oil

Instructions:

- Melt the cocoa butter in a double boiler.
- Add the castor oil, almond oil, and chamomile essential oil.
- Pour into a container and allow it to solidify.
- Apply after a shower to lock in moisture.

Anti-Blemish Spot Treatment

Ingredients:

- 1 teaspoon of castor oil
- 1 teaspoon of witch hazel
- 2 drops of tea tree essential oil

Instructions:

- Mix the ingredients in a small dropper bottle.
- Apply a drop directly onto blemishes and leave overnight.

Hand and Foot Balm

Ingredients:

- 2 tablespoons of castor oil
- 2 tablespoons of shea butter

- 1 tablespoon of beeswax
- 5 drops of peppermint essential oil

Instructions:

- Melt the shea butter and beeswax in a double boiler.
- Stir in the castor oil and peppermint essential oil.
- Pour into a container and allow to cool.
- Apply generously to hands and feet before bed, covering with socks or gloves for deep hydration.

Calming Face Mist

Ingredients:

- 1 cup of distilled water
- 1 tablespoon of castor oil
- 1 tablespoon of rose water
- A few drops of lavender essential oil

Instructions:

- Combine all ingredients in a spray bottle and shake well.
- Mist over your face throughout the day for hydration and a calming effect.

These recipes utilize the nourishing qualities of castor oil to provide a healthy, beautiful complexion while offering an all-natural, efficient method of skin care.

Hair and Scalp Masks for All Hair Types

Castor oil is renowned for its ability to moisturize the scalp, promote hair growth, and generally contribute to the health and beauty of hair. Regardless of whether one has fine, damaged, greasy, or dry hair, there is something in castor oil treatments that can help. The following shows a selection of hair masks and scalp treatments applicable to various hair types and needs.

Deep Conditioning Hair Mask for Dry, Damaged Hair

Ingredients:

- 2 tablespoons of castor oil
- 1 tablespoon of coconut oil
- 1 tablespoon of honey
- 1 egg yolk

Instructions:

- Mix all the ingredients until well combined.
- Apply the mask to damp hair, focusing on the ends and damaged areas.
- Cover your hair with a shower cap and leave on for 30-45 minutes.
- Rinse thoroughly with warm water and shampoo as usual.

Scalp Treatment for Dandruff

Ingredients:

- 2 tablespoons of castor oil
- 1 tablespoon of jojoba oil
- 5 drops of tea tree essential oil

Instructions:

- Combine the oils in a small bowl.
- Apply directly to the scalp and massage in for 5-10 minutes.

- Leave on for at least 30 minutes, then wash your hair as usual.
- Repeat 2-3 times a week to reduce dandruff and soothe the scalp.

Volumizing Hair Mask for Fine Hair

Ingredients:

- 2 tablespoons of castor oil
- 1 tablespoon of aloe vera gel
- 1 tablespoon of apple cider vinegar

Instructions:

- Mix the ingredients until smooth.
- Apply the mask to your scalp and roots, then work through to the ends.
- Leave on for 20-30 minutes, then rinse and shampoo.

Hair Growth Stimulating Mask

Ingredients:

- 2 tablespoons of castor oil
- 1 tablespoon of onion juice (rich in sulfur to boost hair growth)
- 1 tablespoon of coconut milk (nourishing for the scalp)

Instructions:

- Combine the ingredients in a bowl.
- Apply the mixture to your scalp and massage gently.
- Leave on for 30 minutes, then rinse thoroughly and wash your hair with a mild shampoo.

- Use weekly for best results.

Repairing Mask for Chemically Treated Hair

Ingredients:

- 2 tablespoons of castor oil
- 1 tablespoon of avocado oil
- 1 tablespoon of shea butter (melted)
- A few drops of rosemary essential oil

Instructions:

- Mix all the ingredients into a smooth paste.
- Apply generously to the hair, focusing on the areas that have been damaged by chemical treatments.
- Leave on for 45 minutes, then rinse and shampoo.

Balancing Mask for Oily Hair

Ingredients:

- 2 tablespoons of castor oil
- 1 tablespoon of lemon juice (natural astringent)
- 1 tablespoon of aloe vera gel

Instructions:

- Mix the ingredients until smooth.
- Apply the mask to the scalp and roots, avoiding the ends if they are not oily.
- Leave on for 15-20 minutes, then rinse and wash your hair with a clarifying shampoo.

Nourishing Leave-In Conditioner

Ingredients:

- 1 tablespoon of castor oil
- 1 tablespoon of argan oil
- 1 tablespoon of distilled water
- A few drops of lavender essential oil

Instructions:

- Mix all ingredients in a spray bottle and shake well.
- Lightly spray on damp hair, focusing on the ends to nourish and protect without weighing hair down.

Frizz Control Serum

Ingredients:

- 1 tablespoon of castor oil
- 1 tablespoon of grapeseed oil (lightweight and non-greasy)
- 1 tablespoon of aloe vera gel

Instructions:

- Combine the ingredients and apply a small amount to damp or dry hair, focusing on frizzy areas.
- Style as usual.

Overnight Hair Repair Treatment

Ingredients:

- 2 tablespoons of castor oil
- 1 tablespoon of olive oil
- A few drops of peppermint essential oil (for a refreshing scalp treatment)

Instructions:

- Mix the oils and apply to your hair before bed, focusing on damaged areas.
- Cover with a shower cap or silk scarf and leave overnight.
- Wash out in the morning with a gentle shampoo.

Anti-Hair Loss Treatment

Ingredients:

- 2 tablespoons of castor oil
- 1 tablespoon of rosemary essential oil (known for promoting hair growth)
- 1 tablespoon of almond oil (for added nourishment)

Instructions:

- Mix all ingredients and apply to the scalp and roots.
- Massage for 5-10 minutes to stimulate blood flow.
- Leave on for at least 30 minutes, then rinse and shampoo.

They are a natural and efficient way of feeding the hair and keeping the scalp healthy. The treatments can also be done per your unique hair type and needs.

Maintaining Healthy Hands with Cuticles and Nails Using Castor Oil

Another great use for castor oil, along with the other advantages it has for skin and hair, is nail and cuticle treatment. The thick viscosity of castor oil is perfect for giving strength to your nails and hydrating them. Its antibacterial and antifungal properties protect against infections of any kind. With regular use, your hands will look and feel much better, with strong, robust nails and moisturized, smooth cuticles.

Nail Strengthening Treatment

Ingredients:

- 1 tablespoon of castor oil
- 1 tablespoon of jojoba oil (for added nourishment)
- A few drops of lemon essential oil (to brighten nails)

Instructions:

- Mix the oils in a small bowl.
- Apply to your nails and cuticles, massaging in for several minutes.
- Leave on overnight for best results, or rinse after 30 minutes if preferred.
- Use daily to strengthen weak, brittle nails.

Cuticle Softening Balm

Ingredients:

- 2 tablespoons of castor oil
- 1 tablespoon of shea butter
- 1 tablespoon of beeswax (melted)
- A few drops of tea tree essential oil (for its antifungal properties)

Instructions:

- Melt the shea butter and beeswax in a double boiler.
- Stir in the castor oil and tea tree essential oil.

- Pour the mixture into a small container and allow it to solidify.
- Massage into your cuticles daily to keep them soft and healthy.

Nail Growth Serum

Ingredients:

- 1 tablespoon of castor oil
- 1 tablespoon of almond oil
- 1 tablespoon of vitamin E oil (known for its strengthening properties)

Instructions:

- Combine the oils in a small bottle with a dropper.
- Apply a drop to each nail and massage in, focusing on the base of the nail where growth occurs.
- Use daily to encourage faster, healthier nail growth.

Anti-Fungal Nail Treatment

Ingredients:

- 1 tablespoon of castor oil
- 1 tablespoon of coconut oil (known for its antifungal properties)
- A few drops of oregano essential oil (another powerful antifungal)

Instructions:

- Mix the ingredients in a small bowl.
- Apply to affected nails and cuticles, massaging in well.

- Leave on for at least 30 minutes, or overnight if possible, and rinse off.
- Use regularly until the infection clears.

Hand and Nail Cream

Ingredients:

- 2 tablespoons of castor oil
- 2 tablespoons of cocoa butter (for deep hydration)
- 1 tablespoon of almond oil
- A few drops of lavender essential oil (for soothing fragrance)

Instructions:

- Melt the cocoa butter in a double boiler.
- Stir in the castor oil, almond oil, and lavender essential oil.
- Pour into a small container and allow to cool.
- Apply generously to hands and nails daily, especially before bed.

Nail Whitening Treatment

Ingredients:

- 1 tablespoon of castor oil
- 1 tablespoon of baking soda (a natural whitener)
- A few drops of lemon juice

Instructions:

- Mix the ingredients into a paste.
- Apply to nails and let sit for 5-10 minutes.
- Rinse off with warm water, using a nail brush if necessary.

- Use weekly to maintain bright, healthy nails.

Intensive Cuticle Repair Treatment

Ingredients:

- 1 tablespoon of castor oil
- 1 tablespoon of olive oil
- 1 tablespoon of honey (a natural humectant)

Instructions:

- Mix the ingredients in a small bowl.
- Apply to cuticles and massage in thoroughly.
- Leave on for 15-20 minutes, then rinse with warm water.
- Use regularly to repair and hydrate damaged cuticles.

Nail Polish Remover Alternative

Ingredients:

- 1 tablespoon of castor oil
- 1 tablespoon of lemon juice
- 1 tablespoon of vinegar

Instructions:

- Combine the ingredients in a small bowl.
- Soak a cotton ball in the mixture and use it to remove nail polish.
- This natural alternative is less drying than traditional removers and helps keep nails healthy.

Nail and Cuticle Softening Soak

Ingredients:

- 2 tablespoons of castor oil
- 2 tablespoons of warm olive oil
- 1 tablespoon of lemon juice

Instructions:

- Mix the ingredients in a bowl.
- Soak your nails and cuticles for 10-15 minutes.
- Rinse and pat dry, then apply a moisturizer.

Hand and Nail Oil

Ingredients:

- 2 tablespoons of castor oil
- 1 tablespoon of jojoba oil
- A few drops of vitamin E oil
- A few drops of lavender or rosemary essential oil

Instructions:

- Combine all ingredients in a small bottle with a dropper.
- Apply a few drops to your hands and nails, massaging in until absorbed.
- Use daily for soft, hydrated hands and strong nails.

These recipes are all easy to prepare, and you can adjust them according to your needs. The castor oil can frequently be used as a method of continued health and strength for grooming your hands.

Generally speaking, castor oil has several uses for skin, hair, and nails, making it one of the strong bases for homemade beauty care. It will be very helpful in maintaining healthy hair, strong nails, and glowing skin owing to its moisturizing effects, healing capabilities, and strengthening properties. You can fully make use of castor oil to enhance your general health and natural beauty by including these simple applications in your regime of beauty care. Be it for stimulating nail treatments, deep conditioning hair masks, or face cream, castor oil provides the base for efficient all-natural care.

Chapter 8:
Natural Remedies for Pain and Inflammation

Handling Arthritis: A Step-by-Step Process for Joint Health

Arthritis involves symptoms like inflammation of the joints, and a person becomes very uncomfortable due to stiffness. It also affects mobility quite a lot. Hence, most people with this condition look for natural remedies to try and alleviate symptoms while traditional treatments often involve anti-inflammatory drugs and painkillers. Castor oil can offer a holistic approach to arthritis management by containing potent analgesic and anti-inflammatory properties that could be incorporated into daily tasks for extended relief.

Understanding Inflammation and Arthritis

While there are many varieties of different kinds of arthritis, two of the most common types include rheumatoid arthritis and osteoarthritis. Rheumatoid arthritis is considered an autoimmune disease because the body's immune system primarily attacks the joints of the body, causing inflammation and discomfort. Osteoarthritis results from wear and tear between the cartilage, causing friction between bones. Whatever the cause, the relief of pain and an improvement in function require the control of inflammation.

Step-by-Step Treatments with Castor Oil
Warm Castor Oil Massage

Purpose: To reduce inflammation, ease joint stiffness, and improve circulation.

Instructions:

- Warm a small amount of castor oil by placing it in a bowl of hot water or using a microwave for a few seconds.
- Gently massage the warm oil into the affected joints using circular motions. Focus on areas where you experience the most pain and stiffness.
- Continue massaging for 5-10 minutes, allowing the oil to penetrate deeply into the skin and tissues.
- For enhanced effects, apply the oil before bed and cover the area with a cloth to keep it warm overnight.

Castor Oil Pack for Joint Pain

Purpose: To provide deep, sustained relief from chronic pain and inflammation.

Instructions:

- Soak a piece of flannel or cotton cloth in cold-pressed, hexane-free castor oil until it is saturated.
- Place the oil-soaked cloth over the affected joint and cover it with plastic wrap to prevent staining.
- Apply a heating pad or hot water bottle on top of the wrap to enhance absorption and promote circulation.
- Leave the pack on for 30-60 minutes, then remove and gently wipe away any excess oil.
- Use this treatment 3-4 times a week for best results.

Castor Oil and Epsom Salt Bath

Purpose: To relax the muscles, reduce joint inflammation, and promote overall well-being.

Instructions:

- Add 2 tablespoons of castor oil and 1 cup of Epsom salts to a warm bath.
- Stir the water to ensure the oil and salts are evenly distributed.
- Soak in the bath for 20-30 minutes, allowing the warmth and therapeutic properties of the castor oil and Epsom salts to ease joint pain and stiffness.
- After the bath, pat your skin dry and apply more castor oil to the affected joints for continued relief.

Castor Oil and Essential Oil Blend

Purpose: To enhance the anti-inflammatory effects of castor oil with the additional benefits of essential oils.

Instructions:

- In a small bottle, combine 2 tablespoons of castor oil with 5 drops of rosemary essential oil (for pain relief) and 5 drops of lavender essential oil (for relaxation).
- Shake well to mix the oils.
- Apply the blend to the affected joints and massage in gently.
- Use this blend daily to manage pain and inflammation.

Long-term Arthritis Treatment

While these therapies greatly alleviate symptoms of arthritis, a healthy lifestyle is important for long-term management of the disease. Possible ways to reduce arthritic symptoms are through regular bodily exercise, consumption of a proper nutrition-rich diet with foods containing anti-inflammatory nutrients, and having a healthy weight. You will be able to improve your overall life quality and manage your arthritis better when using castor oil treatments in addition to an overall approach.

Applying Castor Oil to Sore Muscles and Tension Following Exercise

Exercise is a part of a healthy lifestyle, but it is usually joined by two sidekick companions: stress and painful muscle inflammation. Sore muscles are the result of tiny breaks in the muscle fibers during exercise because pain and inflammation result while the muscles heal and increase in strength. Though this is normal and needs to happen for the muscles to develop, it can be well managed using castor oil to comfort the imposition.

Benefits of Castor Oil in Muscle Recovery

Anti-inflammatory and analgesic, castor oil is a perfect remedy for the muscles strained post-workout. The topical application of the oil allows it to deeply penetrate inside the muscles, hence aiding pain relief by lessening inflammation and hastening the process of healing. Additionally, improved circulation through castor oil helps in the removal of metabolic waste products responsible for muscle stiffness and pain, like lactic acid.

Post-Exercise Castor Oil Treatments
Castor Oil Muscle Massage

Purpose: To soothe sore muscles, reduce inflammation, and promote relaxation after exercise.

Instructions:

- Warm a small amount of castor oil by placing it in a bowl of hot water or using a microwave for a few seconds.
- Massage the warm oil into sore muscles using firm, but gentle, strokes. Focus on areas where you feel the most tension or pain.
- Continue massaging for 10-15 minutes to help relax the muscles and improve circulation.
- For added benefits, you can mix the castor oil with a few drops of peppermint or eucalyptus essential oil, both of which have cooling and analgesic properties.

Castor Oil and Arnica Gel

Purpose: To enhance muscle recovery by combining the anti-inflammatory effects of castor oil with the pain-relieving properties of arnica.

Instructions:

- Mix 1 tablespoon of castor oil with 1 tablespoon of arnica gel in a small bowl.
- Apply the mixture to sore muscles and massage it in until fully absorbed.
- Use this treatment after every workout to reduce muscle soreness and speed up recovery.

Castor Oil Bath Soak

Purpose: To relax the entire body, relieve muscle tension, and promote faster recovery.

Instructions:

- Add 2 tablespoons of castor oil and 1 cup of Epsom salts to a warm bath.
- Stir the water to ensure the oil and salts are evenly distributed.
- Soak in the bath for 20-30 minutes, allowing the warmth and therapeutic properties of the castor oil and Epsom salts to ease muscle soreness and tension.
- After the bath, gently towel dry your skin and apply more castor oil to any remaining sore areas.

Castor Oil Wrap for Sore Muscles

Purpose: To provide targeted relief for particularly sore or tense muscles.

Instructions:

- Soak a piece of flannel or cotton cloth in castor oil until it is saturated.
- Place the oil-soaked cloth over the sore muscle and cover it with plastic wrap to prevent staining.
- Apply a heating pad or hot water bottle on top of the wrap to enhance absorption and promote circulation.
- Leave the wrap on for 30-60 minutes, then remove and gently wipe away any excess oil.
- Use this treatment after intense workouts or whenever you experience significant muscle soreness.

Preventing Muscle Soreness

Of course, it is always important to take all preventative measures so as not to be in discomfort in the first place, even with castor oil treatments to help deal with aching muscles following exercise. One can minimize muscular soreness and help increase recovery by following the right warm-up and cool-down protocols, drinking enough water, and rest and nutrition. Adding castor oil to one's post-workout can help muscles stay healthy and function at their best following a workout.

Treating Headaches and Migraines: A Holistic Approach

Common health problems like headaches and migraines have a great impact on daily living. Over-the-counter drugs are commonly consumed in an effort to treat symptoms. However, many people seek natural solutions that alleviate their symptoms without the adverse implications of drugs. In the treatment of headaches and migraine, castor oil plays an important role holistic medicine because of its anti-inflammatory, analgesic, and soothing effects, whereby pain is relieved and general well-being is improved.

Understanding Headaches and Migraines

It could be caused by many things, such as strain, stress, dehydration, or sinus problems. Migraines, on the other hand, are a little more complex and usually include light and sound sensitivity, nausea, and extreme pain that throbs. A number of causes contribute to the outbreak of migraine, which may range from hormonal modifications to food, stress, and lack of sleep. It is necessary to take proper care of these ailments in an overall way, considering both their causes and symptoms.

Castor Oil Treatments for Headaches and Migraines

Castor Oil Head Massage

Purpose: To relieve tension headaches and promote relaxation by reducing stress and improving circulation.

Instructions:

- Warm a small amount of castor oil by placing it in a bowl of hot water or using a microwave for a few seconds.
- Massage the oil into your scalp and temples using gentle, circular motions.
- Focus on areas where you feel tension or pain, such as the temples, forehead, and the base of the skull.
- Continue massaging for 5-10 minutes to help relieve the headache and promote relaxation.
- For added benefits, you can mix the castor oil with a few drops of lavender or peppermint essential oil, both of which are known for their headache-relieving properties.

Castor Oil Pack for Migraines

Purpose: To provide deep, sustained relief from migraine pain and reduce the frequency of migraine attacks.

Instructions:

- Soak a piece of flannel or cotton cloth in castor oil until it is saturated.

- Place the oil-soaked cloth over your forehead or the back of your neck, depending on where you feel the most pain.
- Cover the cloth with plastic wrap to prevent staining, and apply a heating pad or hot water bottle on top to enhance absorption and promote relaxation.
- Lie down in a quiet, dark room and leave the pack on for 30-60 minutes, focusing on deep, slow breathing to help calm your mind and body.
- Use this treatment at the first sign of a migraine to help reduce its intensity and duration.

Castor Oil and Aromatherapy Blend

Purpose: To enhance the headache-relieving effects of castor oil with the soothing properties of essential oils.

Instructions:

- In a small bottle, combine 2 tablespoons of castor oil with 5 drops of lavender essential oil (for relaxation) and 5 drops of peppermint essential oil (for pain relief).
- Shake well to mix the oils.
- Apply a small amount to your temples, forehead, and the back of your neck, massaging in gently.
- Use this blend as needed to relieve headaches and migraines.

Castor Oil Sinus Treatment

Purpose: To relieve sinus headaches by reducing inflammation and clearing congestion.

Instructions:

- Mix 1 tablespoon of castor oil with 5 drops of eucalyptus essential oil (known for its decongestant properties).
- Apply the mixture to your forehead, temples, and the bridge of your nose, massaging in gently.
- Cover your forehead and nose with a warm, damp cloth for 10-15 minutes to help open your sinuses and relieve pressure.
- Repeat as needed until the headache subsides.

Comprehensive Ways of Preventing Headache and Migraine

Besides the use of castor oil in treating headaches and migraines, prevention needs to be addressed holistically. If one can recognize and avoid triggers, keep to a regular sleep pattern, drink enough water, and manage stress with yoga or meditation, it will be less frequent and less intense. Adding this oil to your wellness routine will help you feel better and cope with your pain positively.

Castor oil is a potent natural analgesic for pain and inflammation, versatile in its application. From headaches, and painful muscles, to arthritis, there's at least one castor oil therapy that will help improve your health and make you feel better. By applying natural remedies in everyday application, you can take responsibility for managing your pain and inflammation, reducing reliance on medicines, and improving the quality of your life.

Chapter 9:
Target Applications: Acne, Stretch Marks, and Other Uses

Castor Oil and Pregnancy: Healing and Prevention of Stretch Marks

Stretch marks are a common complaint during pregnancy since most expectant moms' skin is stretching rapidly to accommodate their growing baby. These blemishes, which most often appear on the thighs, hips, breasts, and abdomen, can become a painful and insecure area for many women. Helping skin elasticity and moisture will help prevent and heal stretch marks, although heredity also plays a huge role in this aspect. Castor oil can be used to prevent stretch marks and reduce their appearance during and after pregnancy, giving them rich nourishing traits.

Comprehending Stretch Marks

When the connective tissues of the skin are stretched beyond their breaking point, collagen and elastin fibers tear, resulting in stretch marks, also known as striae. This tearing leads to the replacement by scar tissue, initially crimson- or purple-colored streaks that ultimately turn silvery-white. Such markings are more apt to occur when a pregnancy's sudden growth and accompanying hormonal changes compromise the integrity of the skin.

Why Castor Oil Works for Stretch Marks

Deep Moisturization: The ricinoleic acid forms about 90% of the castor oil and is one of the fatty acids responsible for deeply moisturizing the skin. This deep hydration prevents rips and the development of stretch marks since it keeps the skin elastic and flexible. Unlike lighter oils, castor oil hydrates the skin deeply and for an extended period of time-something quite crucial during pregnancy.

Enhancing Skin Elasticity: The high content of fatty acids in castor oil nourishes and moisturizes the collagen and elastin fibers of the skin. It allows the skin to stretch more openly, and the skin develops its natural suppleness with castor oil, thereby reducing the chances of stretch marks.

Promoting Healing and Regeneration: Castor oil diminishes the appearance of pre-existing stretch marks by stimulating collagen production and promoting tissue repair. Its anti-inflammatory action further helps in soothing the skin and reducing irritations related to it.

How to Use Castor Oil for Stretch Mark Prevention and Healing
Daily Massage

Purpose: To prevent stretch marks by keeping the skin hydrated and elastic.

Instructions:

- Warm a small amount of castor oil in your hands and apply it to the areas most prone to stretch marks, such as the abdomen, breasts, hips, and thighs.
- Massage the oil into the skin using gentle, circular motions for 5-10 minutes.
- For best results, apply the oil twice daily, in the morning and before bed, throughout your pregnancy.

Castor Oil and Vitamin E Blend

Purpose: To enhance the skin's elasticity and reduce the appearance of existing stretch marks.

Instructions:

- In a small bowl, mix 2 tablespoons of castor oil with the contents of 2 vitamin E capsules.
- Apply the blend to the affected areas and massage in gently.
- Leave the oil on for at least 30 minutes before rinsing off or leave it on overnight for maximum absorption.
- Use this treatment daily to improve skin texture and reduce the visibility of stretch marks.

Castor Oil and Cocoa Butter Balm

Purpose: To provide intense hydration and nourishment to the skin, preventing stretch marks.

Instructions:

- Melt 2 tablespoons of cocoa butter in a double boiler.
- Stir in 2 tablespoons of castor oil until well combined.
- Allow the mixture to cool and solidify, then apply it to the skin as a rich, moisturizing balm.
- Use daily to keep the skin hydrated and resilient during pregnancy.

Post-Pregnancy Stretch Mark Treatment

Purpose: To reduce the appearance of stretch marks after pregnancy.

Instructions:

- After giving birth, continue applying castor oil to the areas where stretch marks have formed.

- For enhanced results, you can mix castor oil with a few drops of rosehip oil, known for its regenerative properties.
- Apply the blend twice daily and massage it into the skin for several minutes to promote healing and fade the marks over time.

Using castor oil consistently during and after pregnancy can significantly reduce the likelihood of developing stretch marks and help heal any that do form, leaving the skin smooth, supple, and healthy.

Acne Treatment: How to Treat Persistent Skin Issues with Castor Oil

Acne is one of the most prevalent skin disorders. It is a condition that encompasses cysts, blackheads, and pimples that almost anyone of any age can have. It usually is a result of a combination of various causes: inflammation, bacterial infection, clogged pores, and excessive sebum or oil production. But of all acne remedies available, castor oil has been considered a safe all-natural solution to the many causes of acne without the many commercial medications that have their side effects.

Why Castor Oil Works Well Treating Acne

- **Antimicrobial Properties:** The high content of ricinoleic acid is accountable for some of the very strong antibacterial effects that castor oil possesses, which help against Propionibacterium acnes - bacteria responsible for acne. This helps in reducing the outbreak by reducing the growth of germs and stops new pimples from coming up.

- **Anti-Inflammatory Effects:** Almost always, inflammation is associated with redness, swelling, and pain in acne. Anti-inflammatory properties of ricinoleic acid help in the process of healing by reducing inflammation, and soothing the skin, hence its utility in both active acne as well as post-acne redness.
- **Balancing Oil Production:** Castor oil, being an oil itself, does not block pores since it is non-comedogenic. Instead, it manages to regulate the production of oils in the skin, hence fitting for combination and oily skin. Castor oil prevents the overproduction of oils responsible for blocked pores and acne because it regulates the production of sebum.
- **Moisturizing and Healing:** Castor oil is a very good skin moisturizer, and it doesn't leave the skin oily. To facilitate healing and minimize irritation, this oil should be used to provide moisture to augment the skin's natural protective barrier. Since the oil penetrates deep into the skin, the healing action is employed where it is most needed.

How to Use Castor Oil for Acne Treatment
Oil Cleansing Method (OCM)

Purpose: To cleanse the skin deeply while balancing oil production and preventing acne.

Instructions:

- Mix 1 part castor oil with 2 parts jojoba oil (for normal to oily skin) or almond oil (for dry skin).

- Apply the oil blend to dry skin and massage it in for 2-3 minutes, focusing on areas prone to acne.
- Place a warm, damp washcloth over your face to open the pores and allow the oil to penetrate.
- Gently wipe away the oil with the cloth, then rinse your face with cool water.
- Use the OCM 3-4 times a week to keep your skin clear and balanced.

Spot Treatment for Pimples

Purpose: To target individual pimples with the antibacterial and anti-inflammatory properties of castor oil.

Instructions:

- Dip a clean cotton swab into pure castor oil.
- Apply the oil directly to the pimple, ensuring it is fully covered.
- Leave the oil on overnight to allow it to penetrate and work on the affected area.
- Rinse off in the morning with cool water.
- Use this spot treatment as needed to reduce the size and redness of pimples quickly.

Soothing Acne Mask

Purpose: To calm inflamed skin, reduce breakouts, and promote a clear complexion.

Instructions:

- In a small bowl, mix 1 tablespoon of castor oil with 1 tablespoon of raw honey (a natural antibacterial) and 1 teaspoon of turmeric powder (known for its anti-inflammatory properties).

- Apply the mask evenly to your face, avoiding the eye area.
- Leave it on for 15-20 minutes, then rinse off with warm water.
- Use this mask 2-3 times a week to soothe and heal acne-prone skin.

Overnight Acne Treatment

Purpose: To treat and heal acne while you sleep.

Instructions:

- Mix 1 tablespoon of castor oil with 1 teaspoon of aloe vera gel (for its soothing and healing properties).
- Apply a thin layer of the mixture to your face before bed, focusing on areas prone to breakouts.
- Leave it on overnight, allowing the castor oil and aloe vera to work together to reduce inflammation and prevent new pimples from forming.
- Rinse off in the morning with cool water.

You get cleaner, healthier skin and less inflammation, and you will better deal with acne without harsh chemicals by incorporating these castor oil treatments into your beauty routine.

Scar and Wound Healing with Castor Oil: Quick Recovery Techniques

Wounds and scars are simply a part of the healing process, but occasionally, permanent markings may be left on an individual, which many individuals wish to hide. Castor oil works quite effectively for natural wound healing and even reduces scars, as it enhances collagen synthesis, reduces inflammation, and improves tissue regeneration. Whether your skin bears stretch marks, surgical scars, or minor cuts, castor oil will help your skin look and feel better.

Why Castor Oil is Effective for Scar and Wound Healing

- **Promoting Collagen Production:** Collagen plays an important role in skin structure and is useful for giving strength and suppleness to the skin. The body produces collagen to heal wounds on the skin; sometimes, this can develop into scar tissue. Castor oil encourages collagen synthesis to regain the skin's natural structure and avoids scar tissue growth.
- **Enhancing Tissue Regeneration:** With deep penetration, castor oil helps regenerate natural skin tissue from the inside out. Because of this, it also tends to work really well in minimizing the appearance of scars over time, accelerating the healing process of a wound.
- **Reducing Inflammation:** While one would think that inflammation is a normal, healthy reaction to injury, it actually prevents the healing process and increases scarring. Anti-inflammatory properties in castor oil work to soothe the skin, reduce edema, and promote the most favorable conditions for optimal healing.
- **Moisturizing and Softening Scar Tissue:** Scar tissues tend to look different often because of their nature, which is dry, taut, and unforgiving. Castor oil's deeply moisturizing action supports the softening of scar tissue, improving its elasticity and appearance. It is also vital for keeping the skin

hydrated and preventing further scarring from taking place.

How to Use Castor Oil for Scar and Wound Healing
Daily Scar Treatment

Purpose: To reduce the appearance of existing scars and prevent new ones from forming.

Instructions:

- Apply a small amount of castor oil directly to the scarred area.
- Massage the oil into the skin using gentle, circular motions for 5-10 minutes to stimulate blood flow and collagen production.
- Leave the oil on for at least 30 minutes, or overnight for deeper absorption.
- Use this treatment daily for several weeks or months, depending on the size and age of the scar, to see noticeable improvements in texture and appearance.

Castor Oil and Baking Soda Paste

Purpose: To exfoliate dead skin cells, promote cell turnover, and reduce the appearance of scars.

Instructions:

- In a small bowl, mix 1 tablespoon of castor oil with 1 teaspoon of baking soda to form a thick paste.

- Apply the paste to the scarred area and gently massage it in for 2-3 minutes.
- Leave it on for 15 minutes, then rinse off with warm water.
- Use this treatment 2-3 times a week to exfoliate the skin and promote healing.

Overnight Healing Balm

Purpose: To promote deep healing and reduce the formation of scar tissue on new wounds.

Instructions:

- Mix 2 tablespoons of castor oil with 1 tablespoon of shea butter (known for its healing properties).
- Add a few drops of lavender essential oil for its soothing and antiseptic qualities.
- Apply the balm to the wound or scar and cover it with a bandage or gauze.
- Leave it on overnight, allowing the balm to penetrate deeply and promote healing.
- Repeat nightly until the wound is fully healed or the scar is minimized.

Post-Surgical Scar Care

Purpose: To reduce the appearance of surgical scars and improve skin texture.

Instructions:

- Once the wound has fully closed and your doctor has given the go-ahead, begin applying castor oil to the surgical scar.

- Apply a thin layer of castor oil to the scar and massage it in gently for several minutes.
- Cover the area with a silicone scar sheet or gauze to keep the oil in place and protect the scar.
- Use this treatment daily to soften the scar tissue and reduce its visibility over time.

Preventing Scars from Wounds

Castor oil helps not only to treat scars that already appeared but also to prevent others. This minimizes the chance of scarring due to cuts, scrapes, and other traumas via a moisturizing effect with improved body natural healing processes.

Immediate Wound Care

Purpose: To prevent infection and promote quick healing, reducing the risk of scarring.

Instructions:

- After cleaning the wound with mild soap and water, apply a small amount of castor oil directly to the wound.
- Cover the wound with a bandage to protect it and keep it moist.
- Reapply castor oil and change the bandage daily until the wound is healed.

Castor Oil and Honey Healing Gel

Purpose: To combine the healing properties of castor oil and honey, creating a powerful remedy for wound healing.

Instructions:

- In a small bowl, mix 1 tablespoon of castor oil with 1 tablespoon of raw honey.
- Apply the mixture to the wound and cover with a bandage.
- Leave it on for several hours or overnight before rinsing and reapplying.
- Use this treatment until the wound is fully healed and there is no risk of scarring.

You will be able to deal confidently with scars, reduce their appearance, boost rapid wound healing, and maintain resilient, healthy skin once you start incorporating these castor oil treatments into your skincare routine.

In a nutshell, castor oil is a polyvalent, strong natural agent that has several benefits in the treatment and prevention of stretch marks, acne control, and promotion of fast and efficient healing of wounds and scars. Such a unique combination of regenerative, anti-inflammatory, and moisturizing properties turns this oil into a priceless tool for a person willing to improve skin condition and appearance. You will be able to incorporate castor oil into your routine for smoother, healthier, and more radiant skin by using it to perform the curative effects for a variety of skin problems.

Chapter 10:
Digestion and Oral Health

Safe, Natural Remedies for Constipation with Castor Oil

Constipation is one of the most common digestive complaints, characterized by discomfort, bloating, and a feeling of incomplete evacuation regardless of age. Though there are plenty of over-the-counter laxatives available, their administration can sometimes cause electrolyte imbalances, dependence on the agent, or dehydration of the body. In light of its unique properties, castor oil is a nontoxic natural alternative to synthetic laxative drugs that safely relieve constipation without unpleasant side effects.

Conclusion to Constipation

Constipation can be defined as, the standard definition, less than three bowel movements per week. A low-fiber diet, inadequate hydration, inactivity, and some drugs may cause constipation. Treatment of chronic constipation is important to prevent consequences like fecal impaction, anal fissures, and hemorrhoids. Therefore, the treatment needs to be prompt and effective.

How Constipation Is Treated with Castor Oil

- **Stimulating the Intestines:** Ricinoleic acid is an active castor oil ingredient responsible for the laxative effect. Upon intake, ricinoleic acid is naturally released into the small intestine, which naturally initiates an intestinal response called peristalsis- a contraction of muscles. This increased motion pushes the feces through the intestines, promoting a bowel movement.

- **Softening the Stool:** Castor oil facilitates the stool's softening by enhancing the intestines' absorbing ability. Thus, it allows for the easy passage of feces through the colon without putting excessive pressure and pain associated with constipation.
- **Rapid Action:** Castor oil acts very effectively in the rapid initiation of action when used to relieve constipation. It is the best option for quick results since it works within two to six hours after consumption.

How to Use Castor Oil for Constipation Relief

Direct Oral Consumption

Purpose: To stimulate bowel movements and relieve constipation.

Instructions:

- The typical dosage for adults is 1-2 tablespoons of castor oil taken on an empty stomach.
- For children over 2 years old, the dosage should be reduced to 1-2 teaspoons, but it's advisable to consult a healthcare provider before administering castor oil to children.
- Mix the castor oil with a small amount of juice or a glass of warm water to mask its strong taste and make it easier to swallow.
- After consuming castor oil, stay hydrated by drinking plenty of water to aid in the digestive process and prevent dehydration.
- Relief should occur within 2-6 hours, so plan your intake accordingly.

Castor Oil and Lemon Juice

Purpose: To enhance the taste and effectiveness of castor oil for constipation relief.

Instructions:

- Mix 1 tablespoon of castor oil with the juice of half a lemon.
- Lemon juice can help neutralize the taste of castor oil and has its own mild laxative effect, which can enhance the overall effectiveness.
- Drink the mixture on an empty stomach, followed by a glass of warm water.
- Expect a bowel movement within a few hours.

Castor Oil Capsule

Purpose: To provide a convenient and tasteless option for taking castor oil.

Instructions:

- Castor oil is available in capsule form, which allows for easy consumption without the strong taste.
- Follow the dosage instructions provided on the packaging, typically 1-2 capsules for adults.
- Drink plenty of water after taking the capsules to aid digestion and promote bowel movements.

Precautions and Considerations

Though effective, castor oil should be used judiciously to alleviate constipation. This is a potent laxative; excessive use of this medication could be debilitating by leading to electrolyte imbalances and dehydration, eventually making the bowel dependent on laxatives to express itself. The use of castor oil should thus be reasonable and only when necessary. People who have specific medical conditions, pregnant women, and lactating mothers must seek the opinion of a health professional before the use of castor oil to alleviate constipation.

Using Castor Oil to Promote Digestive Health

Castor oil benefits digestive health apart from its laxative properties. Since castor oil is anti-inflammatory, antibacterial, and therapeutic, it acts useful in treating keeping the digestive system in good order. From indigestion and bloating to chronic diseases like IBS or IBD, quite a few digestive issues can be soothed with castor oil treatment.

How Castor Oil Supports Digestive Health

- **Reducing Inflammation in the Gut:** Generally, most gut diseases, including IBS and IBD, are believed to be driven by gut inflammation. The anti-inflammatory properties of castor oil soothe the intestinal lining, reduce inflammation, and promote healing. Hence, it is useful in cases of diseases characterized by chronic inflammation of the gut.
- **Supporting Healthy Gut Flora:** Gut flora must be balanced for healthy digestion and overall well-being. Because of its antibacterial properties, castor oil maintains the right balance of gut flora by controlling the unwanted proliferation of harmful bacteria in the stomach. This may lead to enhanced immunity, better digestion, and reduced chances of gastrointestinal disorders.

- **Enhancing Bile Production:** The liver produces a digestive fluid, bile, which aids the small intestine in digesting lipids. By promoting the synthesis and secretion of bile, castor oil increases the rate at which fats are digested and aids digestion generally. This effect can be very useful for individuals who have issues with digestion concerning fats or problems with the gallbladder.

How to Use Castor Oil for Digestive Health
Castor Oil Packs for Digestive Comfort

Purpose: To reduce inflammation, soothe the gut, and promote overall digestive health.

Instructions:

- Soak a piece of flannel or cotton cloth in cold-pressed, hexane-free castor oil until it is saturated.
- Place the oil-soaked cloth over your abdomen, focusing on areas where you experience discomfort or inflammation.
- Cover the cloth with plastic wrap to prevent staining, and apply a heating pad or hot water bottle on top to enhance absorption.
- Lie down and relax for 30-60 minutes, allowing the warmth and castor oil to penetrate deeply and soothe your digestive system.
- Use this treatment 2-3 times a week to maintain digestive health.

Castor Oil and Peppermint Tea

Purpose: To relieve indigestion, bloating, and gas.

Instructions:

- Add 1 teaspoon of castor oil to a cup of warm peppermint tea.
- Peppermint is known for its digestive benefits, including its ability to relax the digestive tract and reduce bloating.
- Drink the tea slowly after meals to aid digestion and relieve discomfort.

Castor Oil and Ginger

Purpose: To soothe an upset stomach and support digestion.

Instructions:

- Mix 1 teaspoon of castor oil with 1 teaspoon of freshly grated ginger juice.
- Ginger is well-known for its ability to calm nausea and promote digestive health.
- Take this mixture 1-2 times a day to soothe an upset stomach and improve digestion.

Castor Oil for Irritable Bowel Syndrome (IBS)

Purpose: To manage symptoms of IBS, including pain, bloating, and irregular bowel movements.

Instructions:

- Apply a castor oil pack to your abdomen as described above, focusing on the areas where you experience the most discomfort.
- Use the pack daily during flare-ups or 2-3 times a week for ongoing symptom management.
- In addition to the pack, consider taking a small dose of castor oil (1 teaspoon) mixed with warm water or tea to help regulate bowel movements.

Diet and Lifestyle Considerations

Castor oil works wonderfully for digestive health, but it has to be part of a bigger plan that includes dietary adjustments, regular physical activity, and plenty of fluids. Such a diet rich in fruits, vegetables, fiber, and fermented foods keeps the gut healthy and can help avoid common gastrointestinal disorders like bloating and constipation. Furthermore, practicing relaxation techniques like yoga or meditation to overcome stress may positively affect digestive health.

Castor Oil Benefits for Oral Health: Oil Pulling and Beyond

Dental and periodontal health are very interdependent, and they affect not only the teeth and gums but also the digestive tract and other body systems. Moreover, castor oil can be an excellent addition to your dental care routine as it prevents gingival diseases, dental caries, and plaque reduction. The common uses of castor oil in dental care include oil pulling, a general Ayurvedic procedure that involves rinsing the mouth with oil to clear toxins and improve dental hygiene.

How Castor Oil Benefits Oral Health

- **Antimicrobial Action:** The antimicrobial qualities of castor oil aid in preventing the growth of dangerous bacteria in the mouth, which can cause gum disease, cavities, and plaque. Castor oil helps avoid common oral health disorders and supports general dental hygiene by preserving a healthy balance of oral flora.
- **Anti-Inflammatory Effects:** Gingivitis, or gum inflammation, is a common ailment that, if ignored, can develop into more significant oral health issues. Castor oil's anti-inflammatory qualities aid in healing, reducing swelling, and soothing swollen gums.
- **Moisturizing and Healing:** The thick, hydrating texture of castor oil aids in the healing and comfort of dry, irritated oral tissues. For those suffering from ailments like canker sores, gum recession, or dry mouth, this is very helpful.

How to Use Castor Oil for Oral Health

Oil Pulling with Castor Oil

Purpose: To remove toxins, reduce plaque, and promote overall oral health.

Instructions:

- Measure 1 tablespoon of castor oil and place it in your mouth.
- Swish the oil around your mouth for 15-20 minutes, making sure to move it between your teeth and around your gums.

- Spit the oil out into a trash can (not the sink, as the oil can clog pipes).
- Rinse your mouth with warm water and brush your teeth as usual.
- Repeat this process daily or several times a week to maintain optimal oral health.

Castor Oil and Baking Soda Toothpaste

Purpose: To clean teeth, reduce plaque, and whiten teeth naturally.

Instructions:

- In a small bowl, mix 1 tablespoon of castor oil with 1 tablespoon of baking soda to form a paste.
- Add a few drops of peppermint essential oil for freshness and additional antimicrobial benefits.
- Use this mixture as you would regular toothpaste, brushing your teeth thoroughly for 2-3 minutes.
- Rinse with warm water and follow up with a mouthwash if desired.
- Use this natural toothpaste 2-3 times a week for a brighter, healthier smile.

Gum Massage for Gingivitis

Purpose: To reduce gum inflammation and promote healthy gums.

Instructions:

- After brushing your teeth, apply a small amount of castor oil to your fingertips.

- Gently massage the oil into your gums, focusing on areas where you experience redness, swelling, or tenderness.
- Allow the oil to sit on your gums for several minutes before rinsing with warm water.
- Repeat this treatment daily to soothe gum inflammation and support gum health.

Castor Oil Mouth Rinse

Purpose: To freshen breath, reduce bacteria, and promote oral hygiene.

Instructions:

- Mix 1 tablespoon of castor oil with 1 cup of warm water and a few drops of tea tree or peppermint essential oil.
- Swish the mixture in your mouth for 1-2 minutes, then spit it out.
- Rinse with plain water if desired.
- Use this mouth rinse daily or as needed for fresh breath and a clean mouth.

Adding Castor Oil to your Oral Routine

Castor oil should be incorporated into an oral hygiene routine of frequent brushing, flossing, and dental exams to optimize its benefits for healthy oral maintenance. With this in mind, through the same virtue, you can maintain a good smile while avoiding many oral health problems when using castor oil treatments and maintaining proper dental hygiene habits.

Castor oil is one of the most impressive and versatile solutions for dental and digestive disorders. Being organic is great for incorporating dental health into your routine, as an effective assistant in general digestive health, and as a perfect remedy for constipation. Adding castor oil into your routine may be all you need to kick-start a much healthier and fitter you for oil pulling, stomach pain, or maintaining healthy gums. In this, you will learn from the secure and efficient ways of using castor oil, fully applying it to keep the vital processes running in your body, and enabling you to live a healthy life.

Part 4: Bonus Detox and Cleanse Section

Chapter 11:
Castor Oil Detox Protocols

Detoxification is one such important process that helps the organs get to work and enables your body to purge poisons while keeping you healthy as a whole. The liver, kidneys, and lymphatic system are some natural detox mechanisms in the human body that work day and night to keep toxic compounds away from your body. But when diets are poor, chemicals abound in the environment, stress is high, and lifestyles are sedentary, these systems become overloaded, accumulating poisons and losing health. The most useful, all-natural method of assisting the body's detox processes is castor oil, which is well-renowned for its therapeutic and cleansing qualities. This chapter will consider many castor oil detoxification methods to help cleanse the body, boost the immune system, and promote good health.

Benefits of Castor Oil Packs for Whole-Body Detoxification

One of the great ways of using castor oil for its detoxifying properties is in the form of castor oil packs. This old-time remedy uses a cloth; the abdomen is covered and soaked in castor oil. A heating source is then placed over the cloth to increase absorption. The heat of the source promotes the entry of the oil into tissues, stimulating lymphatic flow and circulation that supports the body's natural cleansing process.

Full-Body Benefits of Castor Oil Packs

- **Enhanced Lymphatic Drainage:** Lymphatic Circulation Improved One of the lymphatic system's roles in detoxification is transporting waste products and toxins from the tissues into the circulation for filtration by the liver and kidneys. Castor oil packs provide increased lymph fluid flow to facilitate the elimination of toxins and reduce congestion of the lymphatic vessels, which helps the body fight infection, heal itself, and improve immunological function besides detoxification.

- **Improved Circulation:** Good circulation ensures better nutrition and oxygenation of tissues and removes waste products that may be produced in metabolic processes. The heat from a castor oil pack stimulates blood flow to the application site, thus aiding general circulation and ensuring that the tissues deeply absorb the detoxifying action of the oil.

- **Reduced Inflammation:** Inflammation is one of the frequent body responses to exposure to toxins. If this inflammation is not treated, it may lead to chronic diseases. Anti-inflammatory agents in castor oil can reduce pain, soothe tissues, and initiate healing. Castor oil packs are highly effective for people with diseases that may include inflammation, such as arthritis, intestinal disorders, or skin conditions.

- **Support for Digestive Health:** Due to its proximity to the liver, intestines, and colon- three organs responsible for digestion- the abdomen frequently becomes the site of application for castor oil. Applications using castor oil packs may trigger digestion, reduce constipation and bloating, and improve the body's efficiency in eliminating waste.

How to Use Castor Oil Packs for Detoxification

Preparing the Pack

Materials Needed:

- Cold-pressed, hexane-free castor oil
- A piece of flannel or cotton cloth (large enough to cover the desired area)
- Plastic wrap or a plastic bag
- A heating pad or hot water bottle
- A towel to protect your clothes and bedding

Instructions:

- Soak the cloth in castor oil until it is saturated but not dripping.
- Fold the cloth to a size that will comfortably cover the area you wish to treat, such as the abdomen, liver, or kidneys.

Applying the Pack

Instructions:

- Place the oil-soaked cloth on your skin over the area you want to detoxify.
- Cover the cloth with plastic wrap or a plastic bag to prevent the oil from staining your clothes or bedding.
- Place a heating pad or hot water bottle on top of the plastic wrap to apply gentle heat.
- Lie down and relax for 30-60 minutes, allowing the warmth and castor oil to penetrate deeply into your tissues.

After the Treatment

Instructions:

- After removing the pack, you can wipe your skin with a cloth dampened with warm water or a mild soap to remove any excess oil.
- Store the cloth in a plastic bag for future use; it can be reused several times before needing to be replaced.
- Drink plenty of water after the treatment to help flush out toxins and support the detoxification process.

Frequency of Use

It is recommended to have two to three applications of a castor oil pack a week for general detoxification. If one has another major health problem, like an inflammatory disease or digestive problems, use it more frequently daily. Over time, this can bring about fairly striking improvements in general health and well-being.

Liver and Kidney Detox: How Castor Oil Helps Filter and Cleanse

The liver and kidneys are responsible for detoxifying the body and purifying the circulation from metabolic end products, toxins, and other harmful substances. The liver metabolizes toxins into a harmless form, whereas waste products and excess fluid are filtered by the kidneys and excreted in urine. Supporting these organs is important to ensure general health and good detoxification. Indeed, with its anti-inflammatory and purifying properties, castor oil can be an ally for kidney and liver health.

Supporting Liver Detoxification

Liver Function and Detoxification: The liver is an indispensable part of detoxification, as it deals not only with metabolic waste products but also with chemicals and drugs from the environment. A liver working overtime cannot clean the body efficiently, and the consequence may be a buildup of toxins, leading to several problems. Castor oil may help stimulate liver activity by enhancing bile production, decreasing inflammation, and improving flow to the liver.

Castor Oil Packs for Liver Health

Purpose: To support liver detoxification, reduce inflammation, and promote healing.

Instructions:

- Apply a castor oil pack over the liver area, which is located on the right side of the abdomen, just below the rib cage.
- Follow the instructions for preparing and applying a castor oil pack as described in the previous section.
- Use the pack 2-3 times per week to support liver health and enhance detoxification.

Castor Oil and Lemon Juice Detox Drink

Purpose: To stimulate liver function and support the body's natural detoxification processes.

Instructions:

- Mix 1 tablespoon of castor oil with the juice of half a lemon.

- Drink the mixture on an empty stomach in the morning to stimulate bile production and promote liver detoxification.
- Follow with a glass of warm water to help flush out toxins.
- Use this detox drink 2-3 times a week for best results.

Supporting Kidney Detoxification

Kidney Function and Detoxification: The kidneys should filter out the waste products, excess fluid, and toxins from the blood and excrete them as urine. When good kidney function is maintained, toxin buildup within the body is prevented, hence effective detoxification. Castor oil improves kidney function in three major ways: it reduces inflammation, improves lymphatic drainage, and increases circulation.

Castor Oil Packs for Kidney Health

Purpose: To reduce inflammation, improve circulation, and support kidney detoxification.

Instructions:

- Apply a castor oil pack to the lower back, over the area where the kidneys are located.
- Follow the instructions for preparing and applying a castor oil pack as described earlier.
- Use the pack 2-3 times per week or as needed to support kidney function and enhance detoxification.

Hydration and Castor Oil

Purpose: To support kidney health and promote detoxification by staying hydrated.

Instructions:

- Drink plenty of water throughout the day to support kidney function and help flush out toxins.
- Consider adding a small amount of castor oil to a detox drink or herbal tea to support kidney health and enhance detoxification.

Nutritional and Lifestyle Factors Related to Liver and Kidney Health

Along with using castor oil, an overall diet and lifestyle must also be focused on supporting liver and kidney functions. Whole grains, fruits, vegetables, and lean meats can provide the necessary nutrients that help support detoxification. This will also ease the burden on the kidneys and the liver by abstaining from or reducing the consumption of alcohol, processed food, and sugar. Along with giving a boost to these vital organs, regular exercise, ample water, and stress-reduction techniques like yoga and meditation will boost overall health.

Lymphatic System Cleansing: A Natural Immunity Boost

The lymphatic system is one part of the body's immune system. The lymphatic system circulates white blood cells throughout the body. This system helps to prevent toxins, waste materials, and other harmful substances from building up within the tissues of any injury. A slow or clogged lymphatic system can result in an accumulation of toxins and depressed immunity, along with a number of other health complications. Castor oil is an effective natural remedy for cleansing the lymphatic system and stimulating the immune system.

The Benefits of Castor Oil in Lymphatic Health

- **Stimulating Lymphatic Circulation:** Instead of having a pumping mechanism to circulate lymph fluid, the lymphatic system depends on blood flow and contraction of muscles. Castor oil packs stimulate lymphatic flow by improving blood circulation and encouraging the flow of lymph fluid throughout the body. This relieves toxicity and lymphatic congestion, which in turn enhances the general performance of the immune system.
- **Reducing Lymphatic System Inflammation:** Inflammation of the lymphatic system may lead to lymphedema, enlarged lymph nodes, and other health issues. The anti-inflammatory action of castor oil helps reduce inflammation of the lymphatic system and aids in the normal functioning of the lymph, hence decreasing the risk for various problems.
- **Improved Detoxification:** Castor oil could increase overall detox processes by improving the lymph's capacity to move and eliminate toxins from the body. Aside from improving immune function, this should improve general health and wellness.

How to Use Castor Oil for Lymphatic Cleansing

Castor Oil Packs for Lymphatic Drainage

Purpose: To stimulate lymphatic flow, reduce congestion, and enhance detoxification.

Instructions:

- Apply a castor oil pack to areas of the body where lymph nodes are concentrated, such as the neck, armpits, or groin.
- Follow the instructions for preparing and applying a castor oil pack as described earlier.
- Use the pack 2-3 times per week to support lymphatic drainage and promote overall lymphatic health.

Full-Body Lymphatic Massage with Castor Oil

Purpose: To stimulate lymphatic flow and promote detoxification through gentle massage.

Instructions:

- Warm a small amount of castor oil in your hands.
- Use gentle, sweeping motions to massage the oil into your skin, starting from your feet and working your way up towards your heart.
- Pay special attention to areas where lymph nodes are concentrated, using circular motions to stimulate lymphatic flow.
- Perform this massage 2-3 times a week to support lymphatic health and enhance detoxification.

Castor Oil and Dry Brushing

Purpose: To enhance lymphatic drainage and exfoliate the skin.

Instructions:

- Before showering, apply a small amount of castor oil to a natural bristle dry brush.

- Use the brush to gently exfoliate your skin, starting at your feet and working your way up towards your heart.
- After dry brushing, shower as usual and apply a moisturizer to keep your skin hydrated.
- Incorporate dry brushing with castor oil into your routine 2-3 times a week to support lymphatic drainage and promote healthy skin.

Supporting Lymphatic Health Through Lifestyle

Apart from applying castor oil to the body, one can conduct other activities necessary for the health of the lymphatic system. For instance, an active life, which entails working out at any level, like yoga, swimming, or walking, greatly promotes lymph circulation and prevents lymphatic vessels from congesting. Other essential elements for the support of healthy lymph include having good stress management, a proper diet high in fruits and vegetables, and hydration. Moreover, you can facilitate your body's natural detoxification processes, along with the castor oil treatment, and enhance your immunity in general by incorporating these techniques into your daily routine.

Castor oil is a natural remedy with numerous benefits that provide support for the liver and kidneys, cleaning the lymphatic system and detoxifying the body in return. Adding castor oil packs, massage, and other treatments to your health maintenance program will help you expand the capacity of the body to detoxify itself, increase its immune functions, and promote general wellness in all areas. Castor oil delivers an undoubtedly natural, safe, and effective key to health, whether for improvement in lymphatic flow, providing assistive support for renal and hepatic functions, or merely maintaining a healthy state.

Chapter 12:
Traditional and Contemporary Use of Castor Oil in Medicine

The healing principles of castor oil in Ayurveda and Chinese medicine

Medicinal applications of castor oil, derived from the seeds of Ricinus communis, have been under use for centuries because of its strong therapeutic action. Castor oil, which can balance the body, promote detoxification, and cure a variety of sicknesses, consequently plays a great role in the two oldest and most comprehensive medical systems of the world: Ayurveda and Chinese Medicine. Knowing the theoretical basis for these traditional uses will enlighten one on the multifaceted benefits of castor oil and its potential applicability to modern medical practices.

Castor Oil in Ayurveda

Ayurveda is a more than 5,000-year-old system of natural treatment that originated in India and focuses on the balance of body, mind, and spirit. Castor oil in Ayurveda is named "Eranda", which is valued for its nourishment, detoxification, and purgation properties.

- **Balancing the Doshas:** According to Ayurveda, when three doshas, namely Pitta, Kapha, and Vata, are in the person's hands, good health is achieved. It is of great benefit to balance the Kapha and Vata doshas. Where Kapha has to do with structure and fluidity, Vata has to do with movement and dryness. The heat and unctuous nature of castor oil balances the dryness of Vata and the heaviness of Kapha, which may be instrumental in treating diseases associated with these doshas: inflammation, joint pain, and constipation.

- **Purgative and Detoxifying Agent:** Detoxifying and Purgative Agent: Castor oil, in Ayurveda, is primarily utilized as a laxative- a medication intended to rid the toxins, Ama, from the body. According to Ayurveda, Ama is the poisonous byproduct of incomplete digestion that gathers in the body and causes disease. In effect, the strong laxative effect of castor oil assists in maintaining general health and vigor by eliminating such toxins from the route of digestion. In Panchakarma, it finds its frequent application-an extensive Ayurvedic cleansing and rejuvenation treatment.

- **Joint and Muscle Health:** Castor oil is used to relieve pain in joints and muscles, especially for those suffering from sciatica and arthritis. Massaging the oil onto the skin or using hot compresses opens up blood flow and reduces inflammation to ease the pain. Castor oil is also used to treat vata-related diseases via a treatment called Basti, which is a medicated enema that deeply nourishes and lubricates joints and muscles.

- **Skin and Hair Care:** as stated by Ayurveda practitioners, Castor oil supports healthy skin and hair. Its nature heals and moisturizes; hence, it finds application in treating various skin disorders such as eczema, skin dryness, and wound healing. Fitting into Ayurveda's holistic approach toward health and beauty, castor oil strengthens hair, reduces hair fall, and encourages hair growth in its application toward hair care.

Castor Oil in Chinese Medicine

One of these traditional systems of medicine that has utilized the medicinal properties of castor oil is TCM or Traditional Chinese Medicine. In this traditional system, health is considered a balance between Yin and Yang, besides a smooth flow of Qi, or life force, throughout the body. Castor oil has many uses to help reinstate balance and promote healing.

- **Qi and Blood Flow:** Castor oil in TCM activates the flow of Qi and blood. It, therefore, enables castor oil to be effective in the treatment of conditions that result from stagnation, such as pain, swelling, and menstrual irregularities. It relieves pain, reduces swelling, and improves general vitality by promoting the smooth flow of Qi and blood.

- **Detoxification and Purgation:** As in Ayurveda, castor oil is used for its purgative action in TCM. The herb helps the body rid itself of toxins, particularly those stored in the digestive tract. This aligns with TCM, focusing on maintaining organ and systemic balance to thwart disease processes.

- **Warming and Dispersing Properties:** According to Traditional Chinese Medicine, cold and dampness are associated with stiffness, pain, and digestive disorders. Castor oil is traditionally believed to possess warming properties that make it useful in managing the above conditions. Topical applications of castor oil poultices and compresses are indicated in traditional practice for warming up the body, dispersing coldness, and relieving discomfort.

- **Application in Gynecology:** Menstrual discomfort and uterine fibroids are two gynecological conditions that TCM treats occasionally with castor oil. It is used topically as a warm compress to ease menstrual discomfort related to menstruation or reproductive health concerns, decrease stagnation, and increase blood flow.

- **Integration into Modern Practices:** Although the traditional applications of castor oil in Chinese and Ayurvedic medicine draw on centuries-old wisdom, they are no less in practice today. The concepts form part of contemporary wellness practices with castor oil to cleanse, balance the body, and treat various ailments holistically. Understanding these traditional uses facilitates integration between traditional and modern medicine for holistic perspectives concerning well-being.

Modern Applications: How Doctors and Wellness Experts Use Castor Oil

With time, there has been increased utilization of natural drugs, and castor oil has gained recognition amongst modern-day physicians and health specialists for the multiple applications that it has found. Where the oil itself has been a part of Ayurveda and other traditional medicines for thousands of years, a majority of its applications have only now been supported by current science, due to which these are utilized in different forms of medicinal and health sciences.

Castor Oil in Medical Practice

- **Laxative for Constipation:** Castor oil as a laxative is very ancient. Due to its capability to cause loose stool, doctors often prescribe it for temporary relief from constipation. This is easily available for all seeking natural remedies for constipation, as the FDA has approved castor oil as a safe over-the-counter laxative.

- **Wound Healing and Skin Care:** Castor oil is favored among dermatologists and injury care specialists, as it offers skin problem healing and assists in injury healing. Minor burns, cuts, and other injuries are kept away from infective conditions due to the antimicrobial nature of the oil. The moisturizing properties also help with skin hydration and repair dry skin with cracks. Due to castor oil's ability to keep the wound environment moist and hence allow tissue regeneration, castor oil is also applied in some modern dressings, particularly chronic wounds such as ulcers.

- **Management of Inflammatory Conditions:** According to rheumatologists and pain management specialists, castor oil has proven beneficial for patients experiencing inflammatory diseases such as sciatica and arthritis. Its anti-inflammatory properties reduce the pain in joints and muscles, making it a useful therapy to complement conventional treatments. Various integrative medicine practitioners use castor oil packs as another modality in treatments for autoimmune and inflammatory disorders.

- **Support for Women's Health:** Castor oil also finds its application in modern gynecology for different women's health conditions, focusing on relieving menstrual discomfort and induced delivery in delayed pregnancies, which always happens under medical control. Castor oil is a natural means of inducing labor because it may provoke contractions of the uterus; therefore, it should be taken only on the prescription of a doctor and with extreme caution.

Castor Oil in Wellness and Holistic Health

- **Detoxification and Cleansing:** Castor oil is often incorporated into cleansing programs among naturopaths and natural medicine practitioners. The above discussion mentioned that castor oil packs are commonly applied to cleanse the liver, enhance lymphatic flow, and promote general well-being. Individuals who wish to support their body's normal mechanisms for detoxification should be advised to use these packs as a recurring modality or as part of seasonal detoxification programs.

- **Digestive Health:** Other than the laxative effect, naturopathic doctors and holistic nutritionists prescribe castor oil for gastrointestinal health. It is applied topically to various conditions, such as irritable bowel syndrome (IBS) and inflammatory bowel disease (IBD), to relieve bloating, heal the gut, and relieve digestive pain. Castor oil functions in keeping the digestive system in good working order by its ability to reduce inflammation and stimulate tissue repair.

- **Skin and Hair Care:** Castor oil is highly appreciated within holistic skincare and natural beauty because of its regenerating and nourishing effects. Estheticians and natural beauty experts recommend castor oil for various skin and hair disorders, including acne, scars, dry skin, and hair loss. The oil is found to be extensively used in producing homemade natural shampoo and conditioners, as well as other homemade skin care lotions, for its nourishing, moisturizing, and growth-boosting properties.

- **Emotional and Spiritual Healing:** In some respects, health practitioners have used Castor oil in holistic therapy and energy medicine for emotional and spiritual healing. Castor oil packs can also be used during therapies that release energy blockages or buried emotions to support emotional balance and spiritual health. Castor oil is always preferred in therapies meant to heal the body, mind, and soul since it is warm and nurturing.

Research and Scientific Validation

Most of the traditional applications of castor oil have been justified through data provided by modern scientific studies and have acted to confirm the efficiency of the oil further. Ricinoleic acid is the main active ingredient in castor oil, and studies have shown it to have remarkable analgesic, antibacterial, and anti-inflammatory properties. These studies justify the use of castor oil for chronic pain and skin infections, among many other ailments. Its possible health benefits continue to be researched today because of its effects on immune function, wound healing, and cancer treatment.

Combining Castor Oil with Other Natural Remedies for Maximum Impact

For maximum benefit, castor oil may be combined with other alternative medications. Though castor oil is an excellent alternative treatment by itself, the action can be enhanced by combining many other alternative drugs. This is a synergistic approach where therapy can be more complete, covering various aspects of health and well-being. It is also possible to provide personalized treatments using castor oil in combination with other natural therapies like essential oils, herbal medicines, and nutritional supplements that maximize the therapeutic effect of each component.

Castor Oil and Essential Oils

For Pain Relief: Pain-relieving remedies of a strong nature can be concocted by mixing castor oil with essential oils like lavender, eucalyptus, and peppermint. Castor oil would work well with the sedative effects of lavender oil, peppermint oil's cooling effect, and eucalyptus oil's anti-inflammatory effects to relieve pain and inflammation. The combination effectively addresses tension headaches, tight muscles, and joint aches.

For Skin Health: Mix active essential oils like tea tree, chamomile, or rosehip oil into castor oil for better performance on skin issues such as acne, eczema, or dry skin. Rosehip oil stimulates the renewal of the skin cells, chamomile soothes the inflammatory states, and tea tree oil kills acne-causing bacteria because of its antibacterial properties. Facial treatments with these combinations can be used in form or topical applications.

For Respiratory Health: Chest massages with castor oil can also be performed for respiratory conditions. It improves the health of the lungs by opening up the airways, reducing congestion, thereby reducing cough. It works with essential oils of eucalyptus, peppermint, and rosemary. This combination effectively works against sinus infections, bronchitis, and colds.

Castor Oil and Herbal Remedies

For Digestive Health: The advantages castor oil has for digestion can be further complemented by adding this oil to herbal extracts such as aloe vera, ginger, and turmeric. Turmeric and ginger are anti-inflammatory herbs that support digestion processes, while aloe vera acts to soothe the lining of the stomach, promoting its healing. This combination helps promote healthy digestion and reduces inflammation. It can be used in teas, tinctures, or as part of a detox program.

For Immune Support: Some herbs that have been administered along with castor oil include Astragalus, echinacea, and elderberry; these strengthen the immune system. These herbs will help fortify the immune system, and castor oil helps with the drainage and cleansing of lymph. This combination may work wonders during illness recovery or during cold and flu season.

For Detoxification: Herbal treatments with liver support and detoxification properties include milk thistle, dandelion, and burdock root. These herbs, in combination with castor oil packs, allow the body to clean itself of these toxins and help the kidneys and liver sustain their normal functions. This combination can be taken to continue supporting the body's natural detox processes or as part of a seasonal detox program.

Castor Oil and Dietary Supplements

- **For Joint Health:** Castor oil helps supplements containing glucosamine, chondroitin, and omega-3 fatty acids to complement joint health. These vitamins provide the raw material of healthy cartilage and reduce inflammation, while castor oil supports joint circulation and topical soothing of the joints. This combination may help people who have arthritis or other joint disorders.

- **For Skin and Hair Health:** Castor oil can be emulsified with other nutritional supplements, such as biotin, vitamin E, and collagen, for enhanced skin and hair benefits. Collagen strengthens the skin's structure; vitamin E provides antioxidant protection, while biotin promotes hair growth. It is very convenient because it can be taken as a daily supplement internally and applied topically.

- **For Digestive Health:** Castor oil digestive enzymes and probiotics promote gut health. Digestive enzymes help digest and absorb the material inside the food, while probiotics will help to keep the gut flora going. These vitamins work great when castor oil's anti-inflammatory and laxative properties are taken into consideration; hence, this helps treat digestive issues and gut health in general.

Creating Tailored Treatment Protocols

The course of treatment should be individualized, using castor oil in combination with other natural therapies in a personalized manner for each patient, depending on their needs and desires for health. This allows for a more holistic and successful course of treatment, encompassing many dimensions of health and well-being. Mixing castor oil with other complementary natural therapies may facilitate your health goals, whether detoxification, skin health, or chronic pain management.

Castor oil is versatile and an effective tool in preventive and therapeutic healthcare due to its traditional medical background and many uses today. It also gives a holistic approach to health, using this oil to vitalize the body's 'inner doctor' while enhancing health and vitality-either used by itself or combined with various other so-called alternative treatments. You may fully utilize castor oil to achieve the best health and vitality possible by using the principles behind modern science, traditional medicine, and natural synergistic therapies.

Conclusion:
Your Journey to Wellness with Castor Oil

It is evident as you draw your investigation of castor oil's potent and adaptable qualities to a close that it has much to offer the contemporary world. Castor oil is a unique natural remedy for a variety of health and wellness issues, from assisting in cleansing and lowering inflammation to boosting skin and hair vitality and supporting digestive health. This conclusion offers a road map for incorporating castor oil into your daily routine, summarizes the main advantages, and helps you choose the best products to guarantee the best results—whether you're new to castor oil or looking to expand your knowledge and application.

How to Integrate Castor Oil into Your Daily Routine for Lasting Results

Incorporating castor oil into your everyday routine may be easy and gratifying. You can see long-term advantages and enhancements to your general well-being by implementing this natural treatment into many facets of your wellness and health regimen. Here's how to incorporate castor oil into your daily routine:

Daily Skin Care Routine

- **Morning:** To hydrate your face and start the day off well, use a tiny quantity of castor oil blended with a lighter carrier oil, such as jojoba or almond oil. This mixture can help keep your skin moisturized and protected throughout the day. Those with sensitive or dry skin may find castor oil works especially well for keeping their skin radiant.

- **Evening:** Cleanse your face and remove makeup with castor oil as part of your evening skincare regimen. Deeply cleaning pores, regulating oil production, and providing nourishment to the skin may all be achieved with the oil cleansing technique (OCM). Use a night serum containing castor oil as a follow-up to moisturize and restore your skin as you sleep.

Weekly Hair Care Treatment

- **Deep Conditioning:** Use castor oil to create a deep conditioning mask for your hair once a week. To encourage circulation and hair development, liberally apply the oil to your scalp and massage it. After applying the mask for at least half an hour or overnight, remove it with your normal shampoo. This regimen will strengthen your hair, lessen breakage, and enhance the general condition of your hair.
- **Scalp Treatment:** Putting castor oil directly on the scalp might help people with problems like dandruff or dryness on their scalps and provide a favorable environment for hair development. Apply it once a week or as needed; mix it with essential oils such as peppermint or tea tree for further advantages.

Digestive Health Support

- **Constipation Relief:** Castor oil is a natural laxative that you may want to try if you have occasional constipation. On an empty stomach, sip some warm water and take one or two teaspoons of castor oil. Since castor oil usually takes effect in two to six hours, plan to remain close to a restroom. To prevent reliance, use this medicine infrequently and only when essential.

- **Daily Detox Drink:** Add castor oil to a morning detox beverage. Combine half a lemon juice, warm water, and one teaspoon of castor oil. This combination has the potential to aid in liver cleansing, encourage regular bowel movements, and improve digestion.

Regular Detoxification Practices

- **Castor Oil Packs:** Use castor oil packs daily to help general detoxification. To enhance circulation, maintain the health of your liver and kidneys, and encourage lymphatic evacuation, apply the pack to your lower back, abdomen, or liver region. Include this exercise two to three times a week as part of a larger detox regimen, particularly after overindulgence in food or during seasonal changes.
- **Lymphatic Massage:** Give yourself a castor oil massage to activate the lymphatic system and improve the body's natural detoxification processes. You may perform this once a week or as needed, especially if you wish to strengthen your immune system or feel lethargic.

Oral Health Maintenance

- **Oil Pulling:** Use castor oil to begin your day with oil pulling. After 15 to 20 minutes of swishing 1 tablespoon of castor oil around your mouth, spit it out and give your mouth a good rinse. This procedure improves oral health by removing toxins and reducing plaque. Make oil pulling a part of your morning ritual to keep your mouth healthy and clean.

Joint and Muscle Care

- **Pain Relief:** Castor oil is used to remedy some instances of joint and muscle pains through topical application. Massaging the oil deep into the affected area can reduce inflammation and alleviate pain. In instances of chronic pain conditions, such as arthritis, try using castor oil packs on your joints several times a week to improve mobility and reduce pain altogether.
- **Post-Exercise Recovery:** Rub castor oil on sore muscles after a strenuous workout to help your body recover. Its anti-inflammatory action may help reduce muscle soreness and quicken the healing process enough to keep you active-continued and pain-free.

By continuing to apply castor oil in the daily and weekly routines, you will be ensuring the perpetuity of many benefits associated with it, extending into various aspects of your health and wellness.

Key Takeaways: The Most Important Benefits of Castor Oil

We have examined the various applications of castor oil for wellness, beauty, and health throughout this book. The following main conclusions draw attention to the most significant advantages of castor oil:

Natural Detoxification and Cleansing

- A potent natural detoxifier, castor oil aids in the body's removal of pollutants. This oil supports general detoxification and well-being by cleansing the liver, kidneys, and lymphatic system, whether used physically in castor oil packs or ingested for digestive health.

Skin and Hair Health

- Castor oil is a great option for skincare and haircare because of its hydrating, anti-inflammatory, and antibacterial qualities. It is a flexible addition to your cosmetic regimen since it helps moisturize dry skin, minimize acne, lessen scars, and encourage hair development.

Pain and Inflammation Relief

- Castor oil is useful in lowering pain and inflammation in arthritis, muscular discomfort, and joint pain because of its strong anti-inflammatory properties. Frequent use can increase overall quality of life, decrease pain, and improve mobility.

Digestive Health Support

- A well-known natural constipation cure that works quickly and effectively is castor oil. Lowering inflammation, encouraging regular bowel movements, and bolstering the liver and gallbladder function also improve the digestive system's general health.

Immune System Boost

- Castor oil strengthens the immune system by encouraging detoxification and lymphatic drainage. Frequent usage can improve the body's defenses against infections, reduce inflammation, and preserve ideal health.

Versatility in Traditional and Modern Medicine

- For ages, ancient medicinal systems like Ayurveda and Chinese medicine have utilized castor oil, and contemporary medical and wellness practices have come to acknowledge its efficacy. It is an important therapeutic and preventative healthcare tool because of its many uses.

These important advantages highlight the significance of castor oil as a holistic treatment that may be utilized to promote a variety of health and well-being objectives. Whether you want to manage pain, cleanse, improve the health of your skin and hair's health, or improve your digestive system's condition, castor oil offers a safe, practical alternative.

Where to Source the Best Castor Oil: What to Look for in Quality Products

Selected high-quality castor oil is essential to reaping the full advantages of its use. Not all castor oils are made equal, and an oil's efficacy can be greatly impacted by its quality. When searching for the best castor oil, keep the following in mind:

Cold-Pressed and Hexane-Free

- **Cold-Pressed:** Seek castor oil that has undergone a cold-pressing process, eliminating the need for heat during extraction. Cold pressing keeps the oil's natural ingredients intact and guarantees that its medicinal qualities don't change.
- **Hexane-Free:** Hexane and other solvents are used to extract some commercial castor oils, which may leave behind chemical residues. Use castor oil without hexane to guarantee a pure, natural product and prevent possible exposure to hazardous chemicals.

Organic and Non-GMO

- **Organic:** Castor seeds cultivated without artificial fertilizers, herbicides, or pesticides make organic castor oil. This encourages ecologically friendly farming methods in addition to a healthier product. Look for certificates like USDA Organic to confirm that the oil satisfies organic requirements.
- **Non-GMO:** Genetically unmodified seeds are used to make non-GMO castor oil. Selecting non-GMO goods lowers the chance of coming into contact with genetically modified organisms and supports organic agricultural methods.

Cold-Pressed Castor Oil Varieties

- **Jamaican Black Castor Oil:** This well-liked kind is distinguished by its strong scent and rich color. It is created by roasting the castor seeds before the oil is extracted, giving it a special composition that is advantageous for healthy scalps and hair development. Look for cold-pressed, premium organic seeds for Jamaican Black Castor Oil.

- **Standard Cold-Pressed Castor Oil:** Compared to Jamaican Black Castor Oil, Standard Cold-Pressed Castor Oil is gentler smelling and has a lighter tint. It is adaptable and useful for many things, including digestive health and skincare. For optimal effects, ensure the oil is cold-pressed and derived from organic, non-GMO seeds.

Packaging and Storage

- **Dark Glass Bottles:** To prevent light and air from deteriorating the oil's quality over time, castor oil should be kept in dark glass bottles. Amber or cobalt blue are the best bottles to keep the oil's potency and prolong its shelf life.
- **Proper Storage:** Keep your castor oil from the direct sun and heat. Instead, keep it somewhere cold and dark. This keeps the oil effective and fresher for extended periods.

Trusted Brands and Suppliers

- **Reputable Brands:** Select Castor Oil from firms with a transparent sourcing and production process. Seek out firms that value their oil's sustainability, quality, and purity highly and offer comprehensive information about the manufacturing process.
- **Customer Reviews:** Examining consumer feedback might give you important information about the castor oil caliber you are considering. Seek for goods that have received great feedback highlighting the oil's quality, purity, and efficacy.

Certifications and Testing

- **Third-Party Testing:** To guarantee purity, potency, and safety, certain premium castor oils undergo testing by independent labs. These tests may verify that the oil lacks impurities like solvents, heavy metals, and pesticides, giving you confidence in the product's purity.
- **Certifications:** Certain items may have additional certifications, such as cruelty-free or fair trade, which attest to ethical and sustainable manufacturing methods, in addition to organic and non-GMO certifications.

Selecting a premium castor oil that satisfies these requirements will help you ensure you're obtaining the best product possible for your needs in terms of health and fitness. Purchasing high-quality castor oil will enable you to take advantage of all the many advantages this adaptable oil offers.

Embracing Castor Oil for Lifelong Wellness

Castor oil is an amazing natural medicine with a long history and various contemporary uses. Castor oil provides a comprehensive, efficient treatment for various health issues, including pain management, skin and hair health, detoxification, and support for digestive health. You may take advantage of castor oil's potent health advantages and encourage a thriving, balanced life by including it in your daily routine.

As you go with your castor oil adventure, remember to select premium items, try various uses, and pay attention to your body's demands. Castor oil may be a useful ally in your quest for lifetime well-being if you use it consistently and with care, assisting you in reaching your health objectives sustainably and naturally.

Castor oil will help you achieve long-term health, vigor, and happiness on your wellness path.

Bonuses

Bonus 1: Quick Fixes for Common Skin Issues

Quick Fixes for Common Skin Issues

Skin issues can arise at any time, often when we least expect them. From sunburns to insect bites, minor cuts, and dry patches, these common skin problems can be both uncomfortable and unsightly. While there are many over-the-counter treatments available, natural remedies offer a gentle, effective, and often more economical solution. Castor oil, with its rich, emollient properties and natural healing abilities, is a versatile remedy that can be used in a variety of quick fixes to address these everyday skin issues. Below, we delve into several practical applications of castor oil that you can easily prepare and use to maintain healthy, radiant skin.

Sunburn Relief Gel

Why It Works

Sunburns are a common issue, especially after prolonged exposure to the sun without adequate protection. The skin becomes red, painful, and sometimes even blistered. Castor oil is an excellent remedy for sunburn due to its anti-inflammatory and moisturizing properties. When combined with aloe vera, known for its cooling and soothing effects, and peppermint oil, which provides a refreshing sensation, this gel can offer immediate relief from the discomfort of sunburn.

Benefits

- **Reduces Inflammation:** Castor oil's anti-inflammatory properties help to reduce the redness and swelling associated with sunburn.
- **Moisturizes Deeply:** The rich emollient nature of castor oil helps to restore moisture to the damaged skin, preventing peeling and promoting healing.
- **Cools and Soothes:** Aloe vera and peppermint oil provide a cooling effect that soothes the burning sensation and reduces pain.

How to Make and Use the Sunburn Relief Gel

Ingredients:

- 2 tablespoons of castor oil (cold-pressed and hexane-free)
- 2 tablespoons of aloe vera gel
- 5 drops of peppermint essential oil

Instructions:

- **Mix the Ingredients:** In a clean bowl, combine the castor oil and aloe vera gel. Stir well until the mixture is smooth and evenly blended.
- **Add Peppermint Oil:** Add the peppermint essential oil to the mixture and stir until fully incorporated.
- **Application:** Apply the gel generously to the sunburned areas. Gently massage it into the skin, allowing it to absorb fully. Reapply as needed throughout the day to keep the skin cool and hydrated.

Usage Tips:

- Store the gel in the refrigerator for an extra cooling effect.
- Use this gel as often as needed to relieve discomfort and promote healing.

Insect Bite Itch-Relief Roll-On
Why It Works

Insect bites are another common skin issue, especially during the warmer months. Bites from mosquitoes, ants, or other insects can cause itching, swelling, and discomfort. Castor oil's anti-inflammatory properties help reduce the swelling and irritation associated with insect bites, while tea tree oil's antiseptic properties prevent infection and further irritation. This roll-on solution is easy to apply and provides quick relief from itching and discomfort.

Benefits

- **Reduces Itching and Swelling:** Castor oil helps to calm the skin and reduce the itching and swelling caused by insect bites.
- **Prevents Infection:** Tea tree oil's natural antiseptic properties help to prevent infection and promote faster healing.
- **Convenient Application:** The roll-on format makes it easy to apply the solution directly to the affected area without mess or waste.

How to Make and Use the Insect Bite Itch-Relief Roll-On

Ingredients:

- 2 tablespoons of castor oil (cold-pressed and hexane-free)
- 10 drops of tea tree essential oil
- A small roll-on bottle

Instructions:

- **Combine the Ingredients:** In a small bowl, mix the castor oil with the tea tree essential oil.
- **Transfer to Roll-On Bottle:** Pour the mixture into a clean roll-on bottle.
- **Application:** Roll the mixture directly onto insect bites to relieve itching and reduce swelling. Reapply as needed throughout the day.

Usage Tips:

- Keep the roll-on bottle in your bag or first aid kit for easy access when you're on the go.
- Avoid using this solution on open wounds or broken skin.

Healing Salve for Cuts and Scrapes
Why It Works

Minor cuts and scrapes are a part of life, but they can be painful and take time to heal. Castor oil's thick, emollient properties create a protective barrier over the wound, keeping it moist and preventing scabbing, which can speed up the healing process. When combined with calendula and lavender oils, this healing salve not only protects the wound but also promotes faster healing and reduces the risk of scarring.

Benefits

- **Promotes Healing:** Castor oil keeps the wound moist, which is essential for faster healing and reducing the risk of scarring.
- **Reduces Inflammation:** The anti-inflammatory properties of calendula and lavender oils help to reduce swelling and discomfort.
- **Prevents Infection:** Lavender oil's antiseptic properties help to prevent infection in minor cuts and scrapes.

How to Make and Use the Healing Salve for Cuts and Scrapes

Ingredients:

- 2 tablespoons of castor oil (cold-pressed and hexane-free)
- 1 tablespoon of coconut oil
- 1 tablespoon of beeswax pellets
- 10 drops of calendula oil
- 5 drops of lavender essential oil

Instructions:

- **Melt the Beeswax:** In a double boiler, melt the beeswax and coconut oil together until fully liquid.
- **Add Castor Oil and Essential Oils:** Remove the mixture from heat and stir in the castor oil, calendula oil, and lavender oil until fully blended.
- **Cool and Store:** Pour the mixture into a clean container and allow it to cool and solidify.

- **Application:** Apply a small amount of the salve to cuts and scrapes, covering the area with a bandage if necessary. Reapply 2-3 times a day until the wound has healed.

Usage Tips:

- Store the salve in a cool, dark place to maintain its potency.
- This salve can also be used on dry, cracked skin to provide deep hydration and protection.

Dry Patch Soother
Why It Works

Dry patches on the skin can be caused by a variety of factors, including cold weather, harsh soaps, or certain skin conditions like eczema. Castor oil's deep moisturizing properties make it an excellent remedy for dry, flaky skin. When combined with shea butter and vitamin E, this soother provides intense hydration and nourishment to even the driest areas, leaving the skin soft and smooth.

Benefits

- **Deep Hydration:** Castor oil penetrates deep into the skin, providing long-lasting moisture and relief from dryness.
- **Nourishes the Skin:** Shea butter and vitamin E work together to nourish and protect the skin, helping to repair dry, damaged areas.
- **Reduces Itching and Irritation:** The soothing properties of this blend help to calm the skin and

reduce the itching and irritation often associated with dry patches.

How to Make and Use the Dry Patch Soother

Ingredients:

- 2 tablespoons of castor oil (cold-pressed and hexane-free)
- 2 tablespoons of shea butter
- 1 teaspoon of vitamin E oil

Instructions:

- **Melt the Shea Butter:** In a double boiler, melt the shea butter until fully liquid.
- **Add Castor Oil and Vitamin E:** Remove the shea butter from heat and stir in the castor oil and vitamin E oil until well combined.
- **Cool and Store:** Pour the mixture into a clean container and allow it to cool and solidify.
- **Application:** Apply the soother to dry patches on the skin, massaging gently until absorbed. Use as needed, particularly after bathing, to lock in moisture.

Usage Tips:

- This soother can also be used as a hand cream or lip balm to keep skin soft and hydrated.
- For an added boost, wrap the treated area with a warm towel for 10-15 minutes after application to help the oils penetrate deeper into the skin.

Anti-Aging Eye Serum
Why It Works

The delicate skin around the eyes is often one of the first areas to show signs of aging, such as fine lines, wrinkles, and dark circles. Castor oil, with its rich content of fatty acids, can help to hydrate and plump the skin, reducing the appearance of fine lines. When combined with rosehip oil, which is known for its regenerative properties, and frankincense oil, which helps to tone and tighten the skin, this eye serum provides a powerful anti-aging treatment.

Benefits

- **Reduces Fine Lines and Wrinkles:** Castor oil helps to hydrate and plump the skin, reducing the appearance of fine lines around the eyes.
- **Brightens Dark Circles:** The combination of castor oil and rosehip oil helps to brighten and even out the skin tone, reducing the appearance of dark circles.
- **Tightens and Tones:** Frankincense oil helps to tone and tighten the delicate skin around the eyes, providing a more youthful appearance.

How to Make and Use the Anti-Aging Eye Serum

Ingredients:

- 1 tablespoon of castor oil (cold-pressed and hexane-free)
- 1 tablespoon of rosehip oil
- 5 drops of frankincense essential oil

Instructions:

- **Combine the Oils:** In a small glass bottle with a dropper, combine the castor oil, rosehip oil, and frankincense oil. Shake well to mix.
- **Application:** Before bed, apply a small amount of the serum to your fingertip and gently pat it around the eyes, focusing on areas with fine lines and dark circles.
- **Massage Gently:** Use your ring finger to gently massage the serum into the skin, taking care not to tug or pull at the delicate eye area.

Usage Tips:

- Store the serum in a cool, dark place to preserve the potency of the oils.
- Use nightly as part of your skincare routine for the best results.

Castor oil is a versatile and powerful natural remedy that can address a wide range of common skin issues. Whether you're dealing with sunburn, insect bites, minor cuts, dry patches, or the first signs of aging, castor oil offers a safe, effective, and easy-to-use solution. By incorporating these quick fixes into your skincare routine, you can maintain healthy, radiant skin and be prepared to tackle any skin issues that arise. The natural properties of castor oil, combined with other beneficial ingredients, provide targeted relief and support your skin's health and beauty, all with the added benefit of being free from harsh chemicals and synthetic additives.

Bonus 2: Detox Your Body with Castor Oil Cleanses

Detox Your Body with Castor Oil Cleanses

Detoxifying the body is a crucial practice for maintaining overall health and well-being. Over time, the body accumulates toxins from various sources, including processed foods, environmental pollutants, and stress. These toxins can lead to a range of health issues, including fatigue, digestive problems, skin conditions, and weakened immunity. While the body has its natural detoxification systems, such as the liver, kidneys, and lymphatic system, these can become overwhelmed by the burden of modern living.

Castor oil, a natural and versatile remedy, has been used for centuries in traditional medicine to support detoxification. Its unique properties make it an effective tool for cleansing the body both internally and externally. In this section, we will explore how castor oil can be used in various detoxification methods, including a detox drink, liver cleanse with castor oil packs, and a full-body detox bath. These methods are designed to help you rid your body of toxins, improve your overall health, and restore your energy levels.

Castor Oil Detox Drink
Why It Works

The castor oil detox drink is a powerful method for cleansing the digestive system. Castor oil has natural laxative properties that help to stimulate bowel movements, flushing out toxins and waste from the intestines. When combined with lemon juice, which is rich in vitamin C and has natural detoxifying properties, this drink helps to cleanse the liver, improve digestion, and support the body's natural detoxification processes.

Benefits

- **Cleanses the Digestive System:** Castor oil helps to stimulate bowel movements, effectively flushing out toxins and waste from the intestines.
- **Supports Liver Detoxification:** Lemon juice helps to stimulate liver function, aiding in the detoxification process and improving overall liver health.
- **Boosts Immunity:** The high vitamin C content in lemon juice supports the immune system, helping the body fight off infections and illnesses.

How to Make and Use the Castor Oil Detox Drink

Ingredients:

- 1 tablespoon of castor oil (cold-pressed and hexane-free)
- Juice of half a lemon
- 1 cup of warm water

Instructions:

- **Mix the Ingredients:** In a glass, combine the castor oil, lemon juice, and warm water. Stir well until the oil is fully mixed with the water and lemon juice.
- **Drink:** Consume the detox drink first thing in the morning on an empty stomach. This allows the castor oil to work more effectively in stimulating the digestive system.

- **Follow Up:** Drink plenty of water throughout the day to stay hydrated and help flush out toxins from the body.

Usage Tips:

- This detox drink should be used occasionally, not as a daily routine. Once a week or once a month is sufficient, depending on your needs.
- Some people may experience mild cramping or frequent bowel movements after drinking this detox drink, which is a normal response as the body eliminates toxins.

Liver Cleanse with Castor Oil Packs
Why It Works

The liver is the body's primary detoxification organ, responsible for filtering toxins from the blood and metabolizing waste products. However, the liver can become overburdened by toxins from processed foods, alcohol, medications, and environmental pollutants. Castor oil packs are an effective way to support liver detoxification and promote overall liver health. When applied to the skin, castor oil penetrates deep into the tissues, stimulating circulation and encouraging the liver to expel toxins.

Benefits

- **Supports Liver Detoxification:** Castor oil packs help to stimulate liver function, encouraging the elimination of toxins and improving overall liver health.

- **Improves Circulation:** The heat from the castor oil pack increases blood flow to the liver, enhancing the detoxification process.
- **Reduces Inflammation:** Castor oil's anti-inflammatory properties help to reduce inflammation in the liver and surrounding tissues, promoting healing and regeneration.

How to Make and Use a Castor Oil Pack for Liver Cleanse

Ingredients:

- 2-3 tablespoons of castor oil (cold-pressed and hexane-free)
- A piece of clean flannel or cotton cloth, large enough to cover the liver area
- Plastic wrap or a plastic sheet
- A heating pad or hot water bottle
- A towel to protect clothing and bedding

Instructions:

- **Prepare the Castor Oil Pack:** Fold the flannel or cotton cloth into several layers and soak it in castor oil until it is fully saturated.
- **Apply the Pack:** Place the soaked cloth over the liver area (on the right side of the abdomen, just below the rib cage). Cover the cloth with plastic wrap or a plastic sheet to prevent the oil from staining your clothing or bedding.
- **Add Heat:** Place a heating pad or hot water bottle over the plastic-covered pack. The heat helps the castor oil penetrate deeper into the tissues and enhances the detoxification process.

- **Relax:** Lie down in a comfortable position and relax for 30-60 minutes while the castor oil pack works its magic. This is a good time to practice deep breathing or meditation to further promote relaxation.
- **Remove the Pack:** After the treatment, remove the castor oil pack and clean the area with warm water and mild soap to remove any residual oil.

Usage Tips:

- Use the castor oil pack 2-3 times a week for best results. If you're new to this method, start with once a week and gradually increase the frequency.
- Store the used cloth in a plastic bag for future use. It can be reused several times before needing to be replaced.

Full-Body Detox Bath
Why It Works

A full-body detox bath using castor oil is an excellent way to eliminate toxins through the skin, the body's largest organ. This method combines the detoxifying effects of Epsom salts, which draw out impurities, with the moisturizing and anti-inflammatory properties of castor oil. The addition of essential oils like lavender or eucalyptus further enhances the detoxifying and relaxing effects of the bath, making it a rejuvenating experience for both body and mind.

Benefits

- **Eliminates Toxins:** Epsom salts help to draw out toxins from the body through the skin, aiding in the detoxification process.
- **Moisturizes and Soothes the Skin:** Castor oil deeply moisturizes the skin, leaving it soft and hydrated after the bath.
- **Promotes Relaxation:** The addition of essential oils helps to calm the mind and body, making the detox bath a perfect way to unwind after a stressful day.

How to Make and Use the Full-Body Detox Bath

Ingredients:

- 1/4 cup of castor oil (cold-pressed and hexane-free)
- 1 cup of Epsom salts
- 10-15 drops of essential oil (lavender, eucalyptus, or your choice)
- A bathtub filled with warm water

Instructions:

- **Prepare the Bath:** Fill your bathtub with warm water. Add the Epsom salts and stir the water with your hand to help them dissolve.
- **Add Castor Oil and Essential Oils:** Pour the castor oil into the bath and add the essential oils. Stir the water again to distribute the oils evenly.
- **Soak and Relax:** Immerse yourself in the bath and soak for 20-30 minutes. Focus on deep breathing and relaxation, allowing your body to absorb the

beneficial properties of the castor oil and essential oils.

- **Rinse and Moisturize:** After your bath, rinse your body with warm water to remove any residual oil. Pat your skin dry with a towel and apply a light moisturizer if needed.

Usage Tips:

- For an enhanced detox experience, drink a glass of warm lemon water before your bath to stimulate the digestive system and promote further detoxification.
- This detox bath can be used once a week or as needed to support your body's natural detoxification processes.

Castor Oil Lymphatic Drainage Massage
Why It Works

The lymphatic system plays a crucial role in detoxifying the body, as it helps to remove waste and toxins from the tissues and transport them to the bloodstream for elimination. However, the lymphatic system can become sluggish due to factors like stress, poor diet, and lack of exercise, leading to toxin buildup and a weakened immune system. A lymphatic drainage massage with castor oil can help stimulate the lymphatic system, encouraging the flow of lymph and the removal of toxins.

Benefits

- **Stimulates Lymphatic Flow:** The massage helps to stimulate the flow of lymph, improving the body's ability to remove toxins and waste products.

- **Reduces Swelling and Inflammation:** Castor oil's anti-inflammatory properties help to reduce swelling and inflammation in the lymph nodes and tissues.
- **Boosts Immunity:** By promoting the elimination of toxins, this massage helps to strengthen the immune system and improve overall health.

How to Perform a Castor Oil Lymphatic Drainage Massage

Ingredients:

- 2 tablespoons of castor oil (cold-pressed and hexane-free)
- A few drops of essential oil (optional, such as grapefruit or lemon, which are known for their lymph-stimulating properties)

Instructions:

- **Prepare the Oil:** In a small bowl, mix the castor oil with a few drops of your chosen essential oil.
- **Warm the Oil:** Warm the oil slightly by placing the bowl in a larger bowl of warm water. Warm oil penetrates the skin more effectively and enhances the massage experience.
- **Massage the Lymph Nodes:** Begin the massage by gently massaging the lymph nodes in the neck, underarms, and groin area using circular motions. Use light pressure, as the lymphatic system is located just beneath the skin.
- **Move Towards the Heart:** Always massage in the direction of the heart, as this helps to encourage the flow of lymph towards the thoracic duct, where it can be returned to the bloodstream.

- **Relax:** After the massage, lie down and relax for 10-15 minutes to allow the castor oil to fully absorb and continue its detoxifying effects.

Usage Tips:

- Perform this massage once a week to support lymphatic drainage and overall detoxification.
- Drink plenty of water after the massage to help flush out the toxins released during the massage.

Castor Oil and Herbal Detox Tea

Why It Works

Herbal detox teas are a popular way to support the body's natural detoxification processes. By combining the benefits of castor oil with detoxifying herbs like dandelion, ginger, and turmeric, you can create a powerful detox tea that helps to cleanse the liver, improve digestion, and flush out toxins from the body.

Benefits

- **Supports Liver Detoxification:** Dandelion and turmeric are known for their liver-cleansing properties, helping to detoxify the liver and improve its function.
- **Enhances Digestion:** Ginger helps to stimulate digestion and relieve bloating, making this tea an excellent addition to your detox routine.
- **Promotes Overall Detoxification:** The combination of herbs and castor oil helps to promote the elimination of toxins from the body, improving overall health and well-being.

How to Make and Use Castor Oil and Herbal Detox Tea

Ingredients:

- 1 tablespoon of castor oil (cold-pressed and hexane-free)
- 1 teaspoon of dried dandelion root
- 1 teaspoon of dried ginger root
- 1/2 teaspoon of turmeric powder
- 2 cups of boiling water
- Lemon juice and honey (optional, for taste)

Instructions:

- **Brew the Tea:** In a teapot or saucepan, combine the dandelion root, ginger root, and turmeric powder. Pour the boiling water over the herbs and let steep for 10-15 minutes.
- **Strain and Mix:** Strain the tea into a cup and stir in the castor oil until well mixed. Add lemon juice and honey if desired for taste.
- **Drink:** Enjoy the tea warm, preferably in the morning on an empty stomach, to kickstart your detox for the day.

Usage Tips:

- Drink this detox tea once a day during your detox period, which can last anywhere from 3 days to a week.
- Combine with a healthy diet and plenty of water to enhance the detoxification effects.

Detoxifying the body with castor oil is a safe, natural, and effective way to support your health and well-being. Whether you're looking to cleanse your digestive system, support liver function, or simply rejuvenate your body, castor oil offers a range of detoxification methods that are easy to incorporate into your routine. By using the castor oil detox drink, liver cleanse with castor oil packs, full-body detox bath, lymphatic drainage massage, and herbal detox tea, you can help your body eliminate toxins, improve digestion, boost immunity, and restore your energy levels. These methods not only promote physical health but also enhance your mental and emotional well-being, making castor oil an invaluable tool in your self-care and detox routine.

Bonus 3: Essential Castor Oil Travel Kit

Essential Castor Oil Travel Kit

Traveling can be an exciting adventure, but it also comes with its own set of challenges, particularly when it comes to maintaining your beauty and wellness routines. Long flights, changes in climate, and exposure to new environments can take a toll on your skin, hair, and overall well-being. This is where an essential castor oil travel kit can be a lifesaver. Castor oil is a versatile, multi-functional product that can be used in various forms to address common travel-related concerns, from dry skin and frizzy hair to sore muscles and jet lag. By creating a compact, travel-friendly kit of castor oil-based products, you can ensure that you always have the tools you need to stay refreshed, beautiful, and comfortable, no matter where your journey takes you.

Hydrating Face Mist
Why It Works

Air travel and exposure to different climates can leave your skin feeling dry, tight, and dehydrated. A hydrating face mist infused with castor oil provides an instant boost of moisture, helping to refresh and revitalize your skin during your journey. The addition of rose water and witch hazel further enhances this mist's hydrating and soothing properties, making it an essential item in your travel kit.

Benefits

- **Instant Hydration:** Castor oil's rich emollient properties help to lock in moisture, preventing dehydration and keeping your skin soft and supple.

- **Soothes and Refreshes:** Rose water and witch hazel provide additional soothing and anti-inflammatory benefits, reducing redness and irritation caused by travel.
- **Portable and Convenient:** The mist is easy to carry and can be used anytime, anywhere, making it perfect for refreshing your skin on the go.

How to Make and Use the Hydrating Face Mist

Ingredients:

- 1 tablespoon of castor oil (cold-pressed and hexane-free)
- 1/4 cup of rose water
- 1/4 cup of witch hazel
- 5 drops of lavender essential oil (optional, for added calming effects)
- A small spray bottle

Instructions:

- **Combine the Ingredients:** In a clean spray bottle, mix the castor oil, rose water, and witch hazel. Add the lavender essential oil if desired. Shake well to combine.
- **Application:** Close your eyes and lightly mist your face with the spray whenever your skin feels dry or tight. Pat gently with your fingertips to help the mist absorb into your skin.

Usage Tips:

- Use the face mist during flights to keep your skin hydrated and refreshed.

- Store the mist in your carry-on bag for easy access throughout your journey.

On-the-Go Hair Serum
Why It Works

Traveling can wreak havoc on your hair, leading to frizz, dryness, and lackluster locks. An on-the-go hair serum made with castor oil helps to tame frizz, add shine, and protect your hair from environmental stressors. The addition of argan oil and rosemary essential oil further enhances the serum's ability to nourish and revitalize your hair, making it a must-have in your travel kit.

Benefits

- **Tames Frizz:** Castor oil's thick, rich consistency helps to smooth down flyaways and tame frizz, even in humid climates.
- **Adds Shine:** Argan oil is known for its ability to add a natural, healthy shine to hair, making it look vibrant and glossy.
- **Protects Hair:** The serum helps to protect your hair from environmental stressors like sun exposure, pollution, and dry air, which can damage and dehydrate your strands.

How to Make and Use the On-the-Go Hair Serum

Ingredients:

- 1 tablespoon of castor oil (cold-pressed and hexane-free)
- 1 tablespoon of argan oil
- 5 drops of rosemary essential oil

- A small dropper bottle

Instructions:

- **Combine the Ingredients:** In a small dropper bottle, mix the castor oil, argan oil, and rosemary essential oil. Shake well to combine.
- **Application:** Dispense a few drops of the serum into your palms and rub your hands together. Apply the serum to the ends of your hair, working your way up to the mid-lengths. Avoid the roots to prevent weighing down your hair.

Usage Tips:

- Use the hair serum before and after flights to keep your hair smooth and manageable.
- Store the serum in your purse or travel bag for quick touch-ups throughout the day.

Travel-Sized Joint Pain Relief Balm
Why It Works

Long flights, car rides, or even carrying heavy luggage can lead to muscle and joint pain. A travel-sized joint pain relief balm made with castor oil provides soothing relief from soreness and stiffness, helping you stay comfortable during your travels. The balm is enhanced with menthol and arnica, both known for their pain-relieving and anti-inflammatory properties, making it an effective solution for any aches and pains you might encounter on the road.

Benefits

- **Soothes Sore Muscles:** Castor oil's anti-inflammatory properties help to reduce muscle soreness and joint pain, providing relief after long periods of sitting or strenuous activity.
- **Provides Cooling Relief:** Menthol creates a cooling sensation that helps to soothe and numb painful areas, offering immediate relief.
- **Portable and Easy to Use:** The solid balm format is easy to carry and apply, making it perfect for on-the-go relief.

How to Make and Use the Travel-Sized Joint Pain Relief Balm

Ingredients:

- 2 tablespoons of castor oil (cold-pressed and hexane-free)
- 2 tablespoons of coconut oil
- 1 tablespoon of beeswax pellets
- 10 drops of menthol essential oil
- 10 drops of arnica oil
- A small tin or balm container

Instructions:

- **Melt the Beeswax:** In a double boiler, melt the beeswax and coconut oil together until fully liquid.
- **Add Castor Oil and Essential Oils:** Remove the mixture from heat and stir in the castor oil, menthol essential oil, and arnica oil until fully combined.
- **Cool and Store:** Pour the mixture into a small tin or balm container and allow it to cool and solidify.

- **Application:** Apply the balm to sore muscles and joints, massaging gently until absorbed. Reapply as needed for continued relief.

Usage Tips:

- Keep the balm in your travel kit for quick relief from muscle and joint pain during your trip.
- Use the balm after long periods of sitting or strenuous activity to prevent stiffness and discomfort.

Moisturizing Hand and Cuticle Cream
Why It Works

Frequent hand washing, changes in climate, and exposure to harsh environments can leave your hands dry and your cuticles cracked. A moisturizing hand and cuticle cream made with castor oil helps to hydrate and protect your hands, keeping them soft and smooth throughout your travels. The cream is enriched with shea butter and vitamin E, which provide deep nourishment and repair, making it an essential item for any travel kit.

Benefits

- **Deeply Moisturizes:** Castor oil and shea butter work together to provide intense hydration, keeping your hands soft and smooth even in dry environments.
- **Protects and Repairs:** Vitamin E helps to repair dry, cracked skin and cuticles, promoting healthy, beautiful hands.
- **Convenient and Travel-Friendly:** The cream is easy to carry and can be used anytime, making it perfect for maintaining hand health on the go.

How to Make and Use the Moisturizing Hand and Cuticle Cream

Ingredients:

- 2 tablespoons of castor oil (cold-pressed and hexane-free)
- 2 tablespoons of shea butter
- 1 teaspoon of vitamin E oil
- A small jar or container

Instructions:

- **Melt the Shea Butter:** In a double boiler, melt the shea butter until fully liquid.Add Castor Oil and Vitamin E: Remove the shea butter from heat and stir in the castor oil and vitamin E oil until fully combined.
- **Cool and Store:** Pour the mixture into a small jar or container and allow it to cool and solidify.
- **Application:** Apply the cream to your hands and cuticles as needed, massaging gently until absorbed.

Usage Tips:

- Use the hand cream after washing your hands or whenever they feel dry to keep your skin soft and hydrated.
- Store the cream in your travel bag for easy access throughout your journey.

Calming Aromatherapy Roll-On
Why It Works

Travel can sometimes be stressful, whether you're dealing with delays, navigating unfamiliar places, or simply feeling overwhelmed by the journey. A calming aromatherapy roll-on made with castor oil and essential oils like lavender and chamomile can help to soothe your mind and body, providing a sense of peace and relaxation wherever you are.

Benefits

- **Reduces Stress and Anxiety:** The calming properties of lavender and chamomile help to reduce stress and anxiety, making your travels more enjoyable.
- **Promotes Relaxation:** The soothing scent of the roll-on can help you unwind and relax, whether you're on a plane, in a car, or at your destination.
- **Portable and Discreet:** The roll-on format is easy to carry and can be used discreetly whenever you need a moment of calm.

How to Make and Use the Calming Aromatherapy Roll-On

Ingredients:

- 1 tablespoon of castor oil (cold-pressed and hexane-free)
- 5 drops of lavender essential oil
- 5 drops of chamomile essential oil
- A small roll-on bottle

Instructions:

- **Combine the Ingredients:** In a small roll-on bottle, mix the castor oil with the lavender and chamomile essential oils. Shake well to combine.
- **Application:** Apply the roll-on to your pulse points, such as your wrists, temples, and behind your ears. Inhale deeply to enjoy the calming scent.

Usage Tips:

- Use the roll-on whenever you feel stressed or anxious during your travels to help calm your mind and body.
- Keep the roll-on in your pocket or bag for easy access throughout the day.

An essential castor oil travel kit is a must-have for anyone who wants to maintain their beauty and wellness routines while on the go. By including a hydrating face mist, on-the-go hair serum, travel-sized joint pain relief balm, moisturizing hand and cuticle cream, and calming aromatherapy roll-on in your travel kit, you can ensure that you're prepared for whatever challenges come your way. These castor oil-based products are not only effective but also compact and convenient, making them perfect for travel. With your essential castor oil travel kit, you'll be ready to stay refreshed, beautiful, and comfortable no matter where your adventures take you.

Bonus 4: Castor Oil Remedies for Pet Care

Castor Oil Remedies for Pet Care

Pets are cherished members of our families, and just like humans, they can benefit from natural, gentle remedies for common health and grooming concerns. Castor oil, known for its rich, moisturizing, and anti-inflammatory properties, is a versatile solution that can be safely used in various applications to care for your pets. From soothing irritated skin to conditioning their fur, castor oil can be an excellent addition to your pet care routine. This section explores several effective castor oil remedies that can help keep your pets healthy, comfortable, and looking their best.

Soothing Paw Balm
Why It Works

Pets, particularly dogs, are constantly on their feet, which can lead to dry, cracked, or irritated paw pads, especially during extreme weather conditions like winter cold or summer heat. A soothing paw balm made with castor oil provides deep hydration and protection for your pet's paws, helping to prevent and treat dryness, cracks, and discomfort. The addition of coconut oil and beeswax enhances the balm's ability to moisturize and protect, making it an essential item for pet care.

Benefits

- **Moisturizes and Heals:** Castor oil's rich emollient properties deeply moisturize dry, cracked paw pads, promoting healing and preventing further damage.

- **Protects Against the Elements:** Beeswax forms a protective barrier on the paw pads, shielding them from harsh surfaces, ice, salt, and hot pavement.
- **Natural and Safe:** This balm is made from natural ingredients, ensuring it's safe for pets if they lick their paws after application.

How to Make and Use the Soothing Paw Balm

Ingredients:

- 2 tablespoons of castor oil (cold-pressed and hexane-free)
- 2 tablespoons of coconut oil
- 1 tablespoon of beeswax pellets
- 1 teaspoon of vitamin E oil (optional, for added healing benefits)

Instructions:

- **Melt the Beeswax:** In a double boiler, melt the beeswax and coconut oil together until fully liquid.
- **Add Castor Oil and Vitamin E:** Remove the mixture from heat and stir in the castor oil and vitamin E oil until fully combined.
- **Cool and Store:** Pour the mixture into a clean container and allow it to cool and solidify.
- **Application:** Before your pet goes outside, apply a small amount of balm to their paw pads, massaging it in thoroughly. Reapply as needed, especially after walks in harsh conditions.

Usage Tips:

- Use this balm regularly to keep your pet's paws soft and protected year-round.

- Store the balm in a cool, dark place to maintain its effectiveness.

Ear Cleaning Solution
Why It Works

Ear infections and irritations are common issues in pets, especially those with floppy ears or those who swim frequently. An ear cleaning solution made with castor oil can help to gently clean your pet's ears, remove debris, and prevent infections. The addition of tea tree oil, known for its antiseptic properties, helps to keep the ears healthy and free from bacteria and fungi.

Benefits

- **Cleans and Protects:** Castor oil helps to gently remove dirt, wax, and debris from your pet's ears, while also providing a protective barrier against infections.
- **Antiseptic Properties:** Tea tree oil helps to prevent bacterial and fungal infections, keeping your pet's ears healthy and comfortable.
- **Soothes Irritation:** Castor oil's anti-inflammatory properties help to soothe any irritation or redness in the ear canal.

How to Make and Use the Ear Cleaning Solution

Ingredients:

- 2 tablespoons of castor oil (cold-pressed and hexane-free)
- 5 drops of tea tree essential oil
- A small dropper bottle

Instructions:

- **Combine the Ingredients:** In a small dropper bottle, mix the castor oil with the tea tree essential oil. Shake well to combine.
- **Application:** Gently lift your pet's ear flap and apply a few drops of the solution into the ear canal. Massage the base of the ear for about 30 seconds to help the solution work its way in. Wipe away any excess oil with a clean cotton ball.

Usage Tips:

- Use this ear cleaning solution once a week to keep your pet's ears clean and healthy.
- If your pet has a known allergy or sensitivity to tea tree oil, you can substitute it with chamomile oil or omit the essential oil altogether.

Fur Conditioning Spray
Why It Works

Keeping your pet's coat shiny and tangle-free can be a challenge, especially for long-haired breeds. A fur conditioning spray made with castor oil helps to moisturize and detangle your pet's fur, making grooming easier and keeping their coat looking healthy and vibrant. The addition of aloe vera and lavender essential oil provides extra nourishment and a pleasant scent, making this spray an excellent all-natural grooming aid.

Benefits

- **Moisturizes and Conditions:** Castor oil helps to keep your pet's fur soft, shiny, and well-conditioned, reducing the risk of matting and tangles.
- **Eases Grooming:** The conditioning spray makes it easier to brush through your pet's fur, reducing pulling and discomfort during grooming.
- **Soothes the Skin:** Aloe vera helps to soothe and hydrate the skin, reducing the risk of dryness and irritation.

How to Make and Use the Fur Conditioning Spray

Ingredients:

- 2 tablespoons of castor oil (cold-pressed and hexane-free)
- 1/4 cup of aloe vera juice
- 1/4 cup of distilled water
- 5 drops of lavender essential oil (optional, for a soothing scent)
- A spray bottle

Instructions:

- **Combine the Ingredients:** In a spray bottle, mix the castor oil, aloe vera juice, distilled water, and lavender essential oil. Shake well to combine.
- **Application:** Spray the solution lightly over your pet's coat, avoiding the eyes and ears. Use a brush or your fingers to work the conditioner through the fur, focusing on areas prone to tangles.

Usage Tips:

- Use this conditioning spray during regular grooming sessions to keep your pet's coat healthy and manageable.
- Store the spray in a cool, dark place, and shake well before each use.

Hot Spot Treatment
Why It Works

Hot spots, or acute moist dermatitis, are painful, inflamed areas of skin that can develop quickly on pets, often due to excessive licking, biting, or scratching. Castor oil, with its anti-inflammatory and antibacterial properties, can help soothe and heal these irritated areas. When combined with calendula oil, known for its healing properties, and chamomile essential oil, which is calming and anti-inflammatory, this treatment can provide quick relief and promote healing.

Benefits

- **Soothes Irritation:** Castor oil helps to calm inflamed skin and reduce itching and discomfort associated with hot spots.
- **Promotes Healing:** Calendula oil aids in the healing process, helping to repair damaged skin and reduce the risk of scarring.
- **Prevents Infection:** The antibacterial properties of castor oil help to prevent the spread of infection in the affected area.

How to Make and Use the Hot Spot Treatment

Ingredients:

- 2 tablespoons of castor oil (cold-pressed and hexane-free)
- 1 tablespoon of calendula oil
- 5 drops of chamomile essential oil
- A small bottle or jar for storage

Instructions:

- **Combine the Ingredients:** In a small bottle or jar, mix the castor oil, calendula oil, and chamomile essential oil. Stir or shake well to combine.
- **Application:** Clean the affected area with warm water and a mild pet-friendly soap. Pat dry with a clean towel. Apply a small amount of the treatment to the hot spot, gently massaging it into the skin. Repeat 2-3 times a day until the hot spot has healed.

Usage Tips:

- Prevent your pet from licking or scratching the treated area by using an Elizabethan collar (cone) if necessary.
- Store the treatment in a cool, dark place, and shake well before each use.

Natural Flea Repellent
Why It Works

Fleas can be a persistent problem for pets, causing itching, irritation, and even allergic reactions. While there are many commercial flea treatments available, they often contain harsh chemicals that can be harmful to your pet's health. A natural flea repellent made with castor oil can provide an effective alternative, using a combination of castor oil and essential oils like cedarwood, eucalyptus, and lemongrass, which are known for their flea-repelling properties.

Benefits

- **Repels Fleas Naturally:** The essential oils in this repellent are known to be effective against fleas, helping to keep your pet free from these pests.
- **Moisturizes the Skin:** Castor oil helps to keep your pet's skin hydrated and protected, reducing the risk of dryness and irritation.
- **Safe and Non-Toxic:** This natural flea repellent is safe for pets and free from harmful chemicals, making it a healthier option for flea control.

How to Make and Use the Natural Flea Repellent

Ingredients:

- 2 tablespoons of castor oil (cold-pressed and hexane-free)
- 10 drops of cedarwood essential oil
- 10 drops of eucalyptus essential oil
- 10 drops of lemongrass essential oil
- A spray bottle

Instructions:

- **Combine the Ingredients:** In a spray bottle, mix the castor oil with the essential oils. Shake well to combine.
- **Application:** Lightly spray the repellent onto your pet's fur, avoiding the eyes and mouth. Use your

hands to work the spray through the fur, ensuring even coverage. Reapply as needed, especially before your pet goes outdoors.

Usage Tips:

- Use this repellent in combination with regular grooming and flea-checking to keep your pet flea-free.
- Store the spray in a cool, dark place, and shake well before each use.

Castor oil is a powerful, natural solution for a wide range of pet care needs. From soothing dry, cracked paws to keeping your pet's coat shiny and flea-free, these castor oil-based remedies offer safe and effective alternatives to commercial products. By incorporating castor oil into your pet care routine, you can help ensure that your furry friend stays healthy, comfortable, and well-groomed. These remedies are easy to make, cost-effective, and gentle on your pet's skin, making them a valuable addition to any pet owner's toolkit. Whether you're dealing with common issues like dry skin, hot spots, or fleas, or simply looking for ways to keep your pet looking and feeling their best, castor oil can provide the natural care your pet deserves.

Bonus 5: Castor Oil for Hormonal Balance and Women's Health

Castor Oil for Hormonal Balance and Women's Health

Hormonal balance plays a crucial role in women's overall health, influencing everything from mood and energy levels to reproductive health and skin condition. Hormonal imbalances can lead to a variety of issues, including irregular menstrual cycles, painful periods, mood swings, fertility challenges, and symptoms associated with menopause. While there are many approaches to managing these conditions, natural remedies like castor oil have gained popularity for their ability to support hormonal balance and alleviate related symptoms.

Castor oil, known for its anti-inflammatory, detoxifying, and circulation-boosting properties, can be an effective tool for women seeking natural ways to manage hormonal issues. In this section, we'll explore how castor oil can be used to support hormonal balance and overall women's health, including methods for menstrual pain relief, hormone-balancing massages, and remedies for benign breast cysts.

Castor Oil Packs for Menstrual Pain Relief
Why It Works

Menstrual cramps, or dysmenorrhea, can be debilitating for many women, causing pain and discomfort that interfere with daily activities. Castor oil packs are a well-known remedy for relieving menstrual cramps due to their ability to improve blood flow, reduce inflammation, and promote relaxation. When applied to the lower abdomen, castor oil penetrates the skin and works to soothe the underlying muscles and tissues, providing relief from cramping and discomfort.

Benefits

- **Reduces Inflammation:** Castor oil's anti-inflammatory properties help to reduce the inflammation that contributes to menstrual pain and cramping.
- **Improves Circulation:** The heat from the castor oil pack enhances blood flow to the uterus, which can help relieve pain and promote the shedding of the uterine lining during menstruation.
- **Promotes Relaxation:** Castor oil packs can help relax the uterine muscles, reducing spasms and easing cramps.

How to Make and Use a Castor Oil Pack for Menstrual Pain Relief

Ingredients:

- 2-3 tablespoons of castor oil (cold-pressed and hexane-free)
- A piece of clean flannel or cotton cloth, large enough to cover the lower abdomen
- Plastic wrap or a plastic sheet
- A heating pad or hot water bottle
- A towel to protect clothing and bedding

- **Prepare the Castor Oil Pack:** Fold the flannel or cotton cloth into several layers and soak it in castor oil until it is fully saturated.
- **Apply the Pack:** Place the soaked cloth over the lower abdomen, just below the navel. Cover the cloth with plastic wrap or a plastic sheet to prevent the oil from staining your clothing or bedding.
- **Add Heat:** Place a heating pad or hot water bottle over the plastic-covered pack. The heat helps the castor oil penetrate deeper into the tissues and enhances its pain-relieving effects.
- **Relax:** Lie down in a comfortable position and relax for 30-60 minutes while the castor oil pack works. This is an ideal time to practice deep breathing or meditation to further promote relaxation.
- **Remove the Pack:** After the treatment, remove the castor oil pack and clean the area with warm water and mild soap to remove any residual oil.

Usage Tips:

- Use the castor oil pack at the onset of menstrual cramps or as a preventative measure during your menstrual cycle.
- Repeat the treatment 2-3 times a week during menstruation for best results.

Hormone-Balancing Massage Oil
Why It Works

Hormonal imbalances can cause a wide range of symptoms, including mood swings, irregular periods, and fatigue. A hormone-balancing massage oil made with castor oil and essential oils like clary sage and geranium can help support hormonal balance by promoting relaxation, improving circulation, and reducing stress—factors that play a significant role in maintaining hormonal health. Clary sage is known for its ability to balance estrogen levels, while geranium helps regulate the endocrine system.

Benefits

- **Balances Hormones:** Clary sage and geranium essential oils are known for their hormone-balancing properties, helping to regulate the menstrual cycle and alleviate symptoms of PMS and menopause.
- **Reduces Stress:** The relaxing effects of the massage, combined with the soothing properties of the essential oils, help to reduce stress, which can positively impact hormonal balance.
- **Improves Circulation:** Massaging the oil into the skin helps to improve blood flow, which can enhance the delivery of nutrients and oxygen to the reproductive organs.

How to Make and Use the Hormone-Balancing Massage Oil

Ingredients:

- 2 tablespoons of castor oil (cold-pressed and hexane-free)
- 10 drops of clary sage essential oil
- 10 drops of geranium essential oil
- A small bottle for storage

Instructions:

- **Combine the Ingredients:** In a small bottle, mix the castor oil with the clary sage and geranium essential oils. Shake well to combine.
- **Application:** Warm the oil slightly by placing the bottle in a bowl of warm water. Apply a small amount of the oil to your lower abdomen and gently massage in circular motions for 5-10 minutes. You can also apply the oil to your lower back and inner thighs.
- **Relax:** After the massage, lie down in a comfortable position and place a warm compress over your abdomen for 10-15 minutes to enhance the absorption of the oil.

Usage Tips:

- Use this massage oil daily or as needed to help maintain hormonal balance and alleviate symptoms of PMS, irregular periods, or menopause.
- Store the oil in a cool, dark place to preserve the potency of the essential oils.

Natural Remedy for Breast Cysts
Why It Works

Benign breast cysts are a common condition experienced by many women, often linked to hormonal fluctuations. These cysts can cause discomfort, tenderness, and anxiety. Castor oil, with its anti-inflammatory and lymphatic-stimulating properties, can be used as a natural remedy to help reduce the size of breast cysts and alleviate associated discomfort. Applying castor oil to the affected area helps to improve lymphatic drainage, reduce inflammation, and promote healing.

Benefits

- **Reduces Inflammation:** Castor oil's anti-inflammatory properties help to reduce the inflammation associated with breast cysts, alleviating pain and tenderness.
- **Improves Lymphatic Drainage:** Castor oil supports the lymphatic system, helping to reduce fluid buildup and promote the drainage of toxins that can contribute to cyst formation.
- **Natural and Non-Invasive:** This remedy offers a gentle, non-invasive approach to managing breast cysts, avoiding the need for surgical intervention.

How to Use Castor Oil for Breast Cysts

Ingredients:

- 2 tablespoons of castor oil (cold-pressed and hexane-free)
- A piece of clean flannel or cotton cloth, large enough to cover the affected area
- Plastic wrap or a plastic sheet
- A heating pad or hot water bottle

Instructions:

- **Prepare the Castor Oil Pack:** Soak the flannel or cotton cloth in castor oil until it is fully saturated.
- **Apply the Pack:** Place the soaked cloth over the affected breast area. Cover with plastic wrap or a plastic sheet to prevent the oil from staining your clothing or bedding.

- **Add Heat:** Place a heating pad or hot water bottle over the plastic-covered pack to enhance the oil's penetration and effectiveness.
- **Relax:** Lie down in a comfortable position and relax for 30-60 minutes while the castor oil pack works. This is a good time to practice deep breathing or meditation.
- **Remove the Pack:** After the treatment, remove the castor oil pack and clean the area with warm water and mild soap to remove any residual oil.

Usage Tips:

- Use the castor oil pack 3-4 times a week until the cysts begin to shrink and discomfort subsides.
- Consult with your healthcare provider before using this remedy, especially if you have a history of breast issues or are undergoing treatment for a breast condition.

Castor Oil for Menopausal Symptom Relief
Why It Works

Menopause marks a significant transition in a woman's life, often accompanied by symptoms such as hot flashes, night sweats, mood swings, and insomnia. Castor oil, when used in conjunction with essential oils like lavender and peppermint, can help alleviate some of these symptoms. Its natural ability to promote relaxation, reduce inflammation, and balance hormones makes castor oil a valuable tool for managing the challenges of menopause.

Benefits

- **Reduces Hot Flashes:** Peppermint oil, combined with castor oil, provides a cooling effect that can help reduce the intensity and frequency of hot flashes.
- **Promotes Relaxation and Sleep:** Lavender oil's calming properties help to promote relaxation and improve sleep quality, reducing the impact of menopausal insomnia.
- **Balances Hormones:** Regular use of castor oil can support hormonal balance, helping to alleviate mood swings and other emotional symptoms of menopause.

How to Make and Use a Castor Oil Blend for Menopausal Symptom Relief

Ingredients:

- 2 tablespoons of castor oil (cold-pressed and hexane-free)
- 10 drops of lavender essential oil
- 5 drops of peppermint essential oil
- A small bottle for storage

Instructions:

- **Combine the Ingredients:** In a small bottle, mix the castor oil with the lavender and peppermint essential oils. Shake well to combine.
- **Application:** Apply the oil blend to your neck, temples, and the soles of your feet before bedtime to promote relaxation and cooling. You can also apply it to the back of your neck or chest during the day to help manage hot flashes.

- **Massage:** Gently massage the oil into your skin, using circular motions to enhance absorption and promote relaxation.

Usage Tips:

- Use this blend nightly to help manage menopausal symptoms and improve sleep quality.
- For hot flash relief, apply the oil blend as needed throughout the day.

Detoxifying Castor Oil Packs for Hormonal Health

Why It Works

Detoxification is a key component of hormonal health. The liver plays a crucial role in metabolizing hormones, and when it becomes overloaded with toxins, hormonal imbalances can occur. Regular detoxification with castor oil packs can help support liver function, improve digestion, and promote overall hormonal balance. By using castor oil packs over the liver area, you can help stimulate the liver's detoxification processes, reducing the burden on this vital organ and promoting hormonal health.

Benefits

- **Supports Liver Detoxification:** Castor oil packs help stimulate the liver's detoxification processes, promoting the elimination of toxins that can contribute to hormonal imbalances.
- **Improves Digestion:** Regular use of castor oil packs can improve digestion and reduce symptoms of

bloating and constipation, which are often associated with hormonal imbalances.

- **Promotes Overall Hormonal Balance:** By supporting the liver's ability to metabolize hormones, castor oil packs can help promote overall hormonal balance and alleviate related symptoms.

How to Use Castor Oil Packs for Hormonal Health

Ingredients:

- 2-3 tablespoons of castor oil (cold-pressed and hexane-free)
- A piece of clean flannel or cotton cloth, large enough to cover the liver area (right side of the abdomen, just below the rib cage)
- Plastic wrap or a plastic sheet
- A heating pad or hot water bottle

Instructions:

- **Prepare the Castor Oil Pack:** Soak the flannel or cotton cloth in castor oil until it is fully saturated.
- **Apply the Pack:** Place the soaked cloth over the liver area. Cover with plastic wrap or a plastic sheet to prevent the oil from staining your clothing or bedding.
- **Add Heat:** Place a heating pad or hot water bottle over the plastic-covered pack to enhance the oil's penetration and effectiveness.
- **Relax:** Lie down in a comfortable position and relax for 30-60 minutes while the castor oil pack works. This is an ideal time to practice deep breathing or meditation.

- **Remove the Pack:** After the treatment, remove the castor oil pack and clean the area with warm water and mild soap to remove any residual oil.

Usage Tips:

- Use castor oil packs 2-3 times a week to support liver detoxification and promote hormonal balance.
- For best results, combine castor oil packs with a healthy diet and regular exercise to enhance detoxification and hormonal health.

Castor oil is a powerful, natural remedy that can play a significant role in supporting hormonal balance and women's health. Whether you're dealing with menstrual cramps, hormonal imbalances, benign breast cysts, menopausal symptoms, or simply looking to improve your overall hormonal health, castor oil offers a safe, effective, and holistic approach. By incorporating castor oil into your self-care routine through packs, massages, and targeted remedies, you can help manage hormonal issues and promote a healthier, more balanced body. These practices not only provide relief from symptoms but also support your body's natural ability to regulate and maintain hormonal health, empowering you to take control of your well-being naturally.

Appendices:

Quick Reference Guides

The concise reference guidelines included herein are very helpful in anybody's use of castor oil for wellness, beauty, or health. These appendices include comprehensive details on typical issues and adverse reactions, simple do-it-yourself recipes, recommended reading and products, and best procedures for storing and using castor oil. These tips can help you get the most out of castor oil, regardless of your experience.

Appendix A: Common Castor Oil Concerns and Side Effects

Common Concerns with Castor Oil and Their Side Effects

While castor oil is safe and effective across its myriad uses, customers should exercise some caution with several of its potential side effects and concerns. In this case, it is possible to ensure that you apply castor oil safely and effectively and, at the same time, help prevent any adverse side effects.

Common Concerns

- **Skin Sensitivity and Allergic Reactions:** Although rare, castor oil does cause skin irritation or allergic reactions among some users, especially those with sensitive skin. Classic symptoms of an allergic reaction include urticaria, swelling, itching, and inflammation. This is why a patch test is recommended before the topical application of castor oil. To ensure you don't have any sensitivity, try putting a small amount of castor oil on a private area of your skin, such as the inside of your elbow, and wait one day.

- **Overuse as a Laxative:** Overuse of castor oil as a laxative may result in electrolyte balances, dehydration, and the development of dependence on laxative administration for normal bowel movements. This oil should be used rarely when the prescription for the dose is maintained. It is not advisable to use castor oil for its laxative action for periods longer than those prescribed without professional medical supervision.

- **Interaction with Medications:** Castor oil can interact negatively with many medications, especially those taken orally or that affect the digestive system somehow. Suppose one is already taking prescription drugs. In that case, it is best to speak with your healthcare professional before taking castor oil internally, especially if one takes it regularly.

- **Use During Pregnancy:** In pregnant women, castor oil is sometimes used to provoke labor. This, however, should only be done under the supervision of a doctor. This is because it can provoke uterine contractions, and pregnant women are normally advised against taking the oil for whatever purpose without the explicit orders of their doctor.
- **Staining and Greasiness:** Castor oil is thick and may permanently stain clothes and bedding. The castor oil leaves a greasy feeling on the skin and scalp. A patient should be cautious about using only a limited quantity of the oil, enabling it to become completely absorbed or, if preferred, wash off entirely. To avoid stains, one should be careful to cover furniture and clothes with towels or plastic wrap before applying castor oil packs.

Potential Side Effects

- **Gastrointestinal Discomfort:** Oral administration of castor oil, mainly in high amounts, can cause nausea, cramps, and diarrhea due to its intense laxative effect. Start with a low dose, gradually increase the dose if one feels the need for it, and ensure hydration to avoid discomfort.
- **Skin Dryness:** While castor oil is well-known for its moisturizing effect, it sometimes causes dry skin if applied too frequently or without dilution with a

carrier oil. If you experience dryness, reduce the frequency of castor oil or combine it with other oils that hydrate well, such as coconut or olive oil.

- **Low Blood Pressure:** Regularly consuming or taking it in large quantities can cause low blood pressure in some people. You should treat castor oil with caution if you have low blood pressure or are on medication to check your high blood pressure. You will also need to consult a doctor if there is a sudden presence of symptoms, like dizziness and the signs of fainting.

- **Electrolyte Imbalance:** It can be used as a laxative too often or in abundance and create an electrolyte imbalance that could impair many of the body's functions. Electrolyte imbalance mediates many body activities, including weakness, disorientation, irregular pulse, and muscle cramping. In particular, if you use castor oil regularly, ensure you maintain an electrolyte-rich diet and take this product infrequently for constipation.

How to Address Concerns and Side Effects

- **Patch Testing:** Always conduct a patch test before using castor oil on the skin or scalp to check for adverse reactions.

- **Proper Dosage:** When applying castor oil, do not continue beyond the recommended period of time without consulting a physician; when used as a laxative, use within the limits.

- **Hydration:** Drink plenty of water with the use of castor oil, especially when consumed, to prevent dehydration and loss of electrolytes.

- **Consultation:** Consult your doctor concerning the use of castor oil if you are pregnant, lactating, or on any medication.
- **Mix with Other Oils:** Use castor oil less frequently or dilute it with other base oils in case you are irritated by it or it dries your skin too much.

Appendix B: Quick DIY Beauty and Health Recipes

Simple Home Recipes Health and Beauty

Due to its versatility and efficiency, castor oil is commonplace in many homemade beauty and health remedies. Here are some fast and easy recipes you can make at home to enhance your hair, skin, and overall care routine.

Nourishing Face Serum

Ingredients:

- 1 tablespoon of castor oil
- 1 tablespoon of jojoba oil
- 5 drops of rosehip oil
- 3 drops of lavender essential oil

Instructions:

- Combine all ingredients in a small glass dropper bottle.
- Shake well to mix.
- Apply a few drops to your face after cleansing, massaging gently into the skin.
- Use nightly to hydrate and rejuvenate the skin.

Strengthening Hair Growth Oil

Ingredients:

- 2 tablespoons of castor oil
- 1 tablespoon of coconut oil
- 5 drops of rosemary essential oil
- 5 drops of peppermint essential oil

Instructions:

- Mix all ingredients in a small bowl.
- Apply the mixture to your scalp, massaging gently for 5-10 minutes.
- Leave on for at least 30 minutes or overnight before washing out with shampoo.
- Use 2-3 times a week to promote hair growth and strengthen hair.

Hydrating Lip Balm

Ingredients:

- 1 tablespoon of castor oil
- 1 tablespoon of beeswax
- 1 tablespoon of shea butter
- 3 drops of vanilla extract (optional)

Instructions:

- Melt the beeswax and shea butter in a double boiler.
- Stir in the castor oil and vanilla extract until well combined.
- Pour the mixture into small lip balm containers and let it cool until solid.
- Use as needed to keep lips soft and hydrated.

Soothing Muscle Rub

Ingredients:

- 2 tablespoons of castor oil
- 1 tablespoon of olive oil

- 10 drops of eucalyptus essential oil
- 5 drops of peppermint essential oil

Instructions:

- Mix all ingredients in a small jar.
- Apply the rub to sore muscles and massage gently.
- Use after exercise or whenever you experience muscle tension.

Anti-Aging Eye Cream
Ingredients:

- 1 tablespoon of castor oil
- 1 tablespoon of almond oil
- 1 tablespoon of aloe vera gel
- 5 drops of frankincense essential oil

Instructions:

- Combine all ingredients in a small container.
- Gently apply a small amount around the eyes before bed.
- Use nightly to reduce fine lines and puffiness.

Healing Cuticle Oil
Ingredients:

- 1 tablespoon of castor oil
- 1 tablespoon of jojoba oil
- 5 drops of tea tree essential oil

Instructions:

- Mix all ingredients in a small dropper bottle.
- Apply a drop to each cuticle and massage in.
- Use daily to keep cuticles soft and prevent hangnails.

Cleansing Oil Blend
Ingredients:

- 1 tablespoon of castor oil
- 2 tablespoons of olive oil
- 5 drops of lavender essential oil

Instructions:

- Combine the oils in a small bottle.
- Massage into dry skin to dissolve makeup and impurities.
- Wipe off with a warm, damp cloth.
- Follow with your regular skincare routine.

Detoxifying Foot Soak
Ingredients:

- 2 tablespoons of castor oil
- 1 cup of Epsom salts
- 10 drops of tea tree essential oil

Instructions:

- Fill a basin with warm water and add the Epsom salts and castor oil.
- Stir in the tea tree oil.

- Soak your feet for 20-30 minutes to detoxify and soothe tired feet.

Moisturizing Hand Cream
Ingredients:

- 2 tablespoons of castor oil
- 2 tablespoons of shea butter
- 1 tablespoon of coconut oil
- 5 drops of lavender essential oil

Instructions:

- Melt the shea butter and coconut oil in a double boiler.
- Stir in the castor oil and lavender essential oil.
- Pour into a small container and allow to cool.
- Apply to hands as needed to keep them soft and hydrated.

Anti-Dandruff Scalp Treatment
Ingredients:

- 2 tablespoons of castor oil
- 1 tablespoon of jojoba oil
- 5 drops of tea tree essential oil

Instructions:

- Mix all ingredients in a small bowl.
- Apply to the scalp, massaging gently to cover the entire scalp.

- Leave on for at least 30 minutes before washing out with shampoo.
- Use weekly to reduce dandruff and promote scalp health.

Appendix C: Best Practices for Storing and Using Castor Oil

Castor oil should be used correctly and in a manner that allows it to maintain functionality and quality. The following are some recommended guidelines to ensure your castor oil works effectively and remains fresh for your health and beauty needs.

Storage Tips

- **Keep It Cool:** Keep castor oil away from direct sunlight and sources of heat, such as a cold, dark place in a pantry or cupboard. Its utility is reduced over time because of light and heat exposure spoilage.

- **Use Dark Glass Bottles:** Amber and cobalt blue, dark glass bottles can protect castor oil from deterioration in light. If your castor oil is in plastic, consider transferring it into a dark glass bottle for better preservation.

- **Tightly Sealed:** Tighten the container properly after use to keep the air out and oxidize the oil. In this way, it will help to extend life and freshness for a longer period of time.

- **Check for Spoilage:** Although castor oil has a very long shelf life, eventually, it will spoil if kept under incorrect conditions. This is spoilage if your castor oil smells rotten, changes color, or becomes cloudy. It's best to replace the oil with a fresh bottle and discard the old one as soon as these signs are experienced.

Usage Guidelines

- **Patch Test:** You'll want to do a patch test before applying castor oil on your skin or scalp, especially if you have sensitive skin. You can check this by applying a small amount of oil at some inconspicuous site, such as behind the elbow, and wait a day to see if any adverse reactions manifest.
- **Dilution:** Castor oil is thick, and hence, it is prescribed to be used with other diluent oils, which could include coconut oil, jojoba, or almond oil. This would be particularly applied to uses related to the skin and hair. Diluted oil may provide better absorption and permeation of the oil all over the skin and hair.
- **Heating Castor Oil:** You may want to warm the oil slightly before applying it for certain treatments, such as deep conditioning hair masks or castor oil packs. Your thistle of castor oil in a bowl of hot water for a few minutes. Heating in a microwave can damage the healthy attributes of the oil and should not be done.
- **Application Tools:** castor oil to particular areas like the scalp, eyelashes, or eyebrows; use clean cotton balls, swabs, or brushes; larger areas like the abdomen or joints, using your hands or a clean towel. Always wash well before and after application.
- **Frequency of Use:** Castor oil may be used daily, once a week, or as needed, depending on what purpose you use it. In skincare and haircare, castor oil should be used two to three times a week. For internal consumption, as in treating symptoms of constipation, take it only when necessary, especially paying attention to the suggested dosage.

- **Cleaning and Maintenance:** In treatments with oil pulling, for example, or castor oil packs, it is best to clean any equipment, clothes, or containers used afterward to avoid accumulation or contamination. Clean these with warm, soapy water, then air-dry before storing.

Safety Precautions

- **Internal Use:** In the case of constipation, the intake of castor oil is done internally, but a recommended dose is supposed to be taken or used and shall not be frequently repeated. It will lead to overindulgence and further dependence, hence other medical problems. In every case, one must consult a doctor before making any internal use of castor oil, especially in cases when one expects or is breastfeeding or there is any already existing medical issue.
- **Pregnancy and Nursing:** It may inhibit nursing and pregnancy, as its stimulative effect on uterine contractions may not make it safe to take in by expectant mothers. Consult a doctor before taking castor oil if one is either nursing or pregnant.
- **Children and Elderly:** The application of castor oil with children and older adults should be done in very small amounts, and great caution should be taken to watch for adverse reactions. One should consult a healthcare professional for appropriate methods and dosage amounts for these age groups.

Appendix D: Resources for Further Reading and Products

The following links provide information and tips for anyone trying to source the best products and improve their learning about castor oil and its uses.

Books and Articles

"The Castor Oil Miracle: Discover the Healing Properties of Castor Oil" by Dr. Joseph Mercola

- Uncover the Healing Properties of Castor Oil" by Dr. Joseph Mercola. This book examines castor oil's numerous health benefits and discusses its conventional and contemporary uses. In this book, Dr. Mercola guides natural health experts in providing helpful guidelines concerning how castor oil should be applied to various medical conditions.

"Edgar Cayce's Guide to Colon Care" by Sandra Duggan

- Sandra Duggan's "Edgar Cayce's Guide to Colon Care" This great psychic and healer, Edgar Cayce, believed a lot in the role of castor oil in healing and cleansing. The book is about the theories of Edgar Cayce regarding the health of colons and the way castor oil packs may be helpful for the proper maintenance of digestive health.

"Ayurveda: The Science of Self-Healing" by Dr. Vasant Lad

- The Science of Self-Healing" Within this book, the reader is introduced to the ideas surrounding Ayurveda, in particular the use of castor oil in Ayurvedic treatments. Dr. Lad discusses how castor oil can address general health and wellness regarding dosha balancing.

"Detoxification and Healing: The Key to Optimal Health" by Sidney MacDonald Baker

- This book covers different detox methods, including castor oil's lymphatic and liver-cleaning properties. It scientifically explains how detoxification pathways promote life extension and wellness.

"The Complete Book of Essential Oils and Aromatherapy" by Valerie Ann Worwood

- Although this book generally deals with essential oils, it is quite helpful since it provides various ways to combine this oil with castor oil to elicit better medicinal benefits. This is a good reference text for those interested in natural remedies and self-formulated recipes.

Online Resources

The Weston A. Price Foundation: (www.westonaprice.org)

- The Weston A. Price Foundation is a great source to learn more about the traditional approach to diet and natural health care. On its website, various articles were published about castor oil benefits: traditional medicine and modern health uses.

Mercola.com: (www.mercola.com)

- Dr. Joseph Mercola's website is one of the best places to look for information on anything related to natural health. Apart from articles, it contains several videos and product recommendations for castor oil and other natural remedies.

National Center for Complementary and Integrative Health (NCCIH): (www.nccih.nih.gov)

- NCCIH conducts and funds research, trains researchers, and disseminates science-based information to the public, healthcare providers, and researchers on complementary and alternative medicine, including castor oil use for a number of health-related issues. This is a well-established website to access information on natural therapies based on scientific research.

High-Quality Castor Oil Products
Heritage Store Organic Castor Oil

- Heritage Store offers a range of premium cold-pressed and hexane-free castor oil products. Their organic castor oil is USDA-certified, while the packaging in dark glass bottles maintains potency. Castor oil packs and applicators are also available from them for convenience.

Sky Organics Organic Castor Oil

- Sky Organics has a bestselling organic castor oil that is cold-pressed, non-GMO, and cruelty-free. It comes in different sizes and is well-suited for skin, hair, and health applications.

Now Solutions Castor Oil

- NOW Solutions has long been a trusted name in affordable, high-quality natural products. NOW Solutions cold-pressed castor oil serves as a versatile castor oil for haircare, skincare, and wellness all in one. It is an excellent choice for those who are new to the use of castor oil.

Jamaican Mango & Lime Jamaican Black Castor Oil

- Morel's product provides pure Jamaican Black Castor Oil, famous for its peculiar processing method and specific properties boosting hair growth and scalp health. It comes in various formulae, such as original, extra dark, and with infusion of essential oil.

Tropic Isle Living Jamaican Black Castor Oil

- Tropic Isle Living is another well-reputed brand indulged in the production related to Jamaican Black Castor Oil. Indeed, their products are widely appreciated for hair growth, scalp health, and several scalp disorders. They sell hair and scalp treatment blends made with castor oil combined with some other natural ingredients.

Suppliers and Retailers

Amazon: (www.amazon.com)

- You will be able to get several types of castor oil on Amazon, whether organic, cold-pressed, or Jamaican Black Castor Oil. It is convenient, as you will also be able to check the products against one another and go through some customer reviews.

Vitacost: (www.vitacost.com)

- Vitacost is an online retailer selling natural or organic products. They sell many different types of castor oil and sometimes give discounts for bulk orders.

Thrive Market: (www.thrivemarket.com)

- Thrive Market is an online membership retailer, offering natural and organic products at a discount. Their offerings of castor oil products include top-rated brands known for quality and sustainability.

Whole Foods Market: (www.wholefoodsmarket.com)

- Whole Foods Market carries various high-quality castor oil products in their personal care and wellness sections. Shopping at Whole Foods allows the customer to physically look at products they are interested in before purchasing and ensures you get a well-known brand.

References

Anjani, K. (2014). *Castor genetic resources: A primary gene pool for exploitation.* Industrial Crops and Products, 62, 109-120.

Asghar, A., & Shakeel, F. (2017). *Castor oil: Properties, uses, and optimization for enhanced bioactivity. Journal of Pharmacognosy and Phytochemistry,* 6(1), 90-96.

Boateng, J., Matthews, K. H., Stevens, H. N., & Eccleston, G. M. (2008). *Wound healing dressings and drug delivery systems: A review. Journal of Pharmaceutical Sciences,* 97(8), 2892-2923.

Kapoor, V. P., & Kalidhar, S. B. (2010). *Medicinal uses of castor oil and castor seeds: A comprehensive review.* Ancient Science of Life, 29(1), 1-9.

Ogunniyi, D. S. (2006). *Castor oil: A vital industrial raw material.* Bioresource Technology, 97(9), 1086-1091.

Patel, V. R., Dumancas, G. G., Viswanath, L. C. K., Maples, R., & Subong, B. J. J. (2016). *Castor oil: Properties, uses, and optimization of processing parameters in commercial production.* Lipids, 51(1), 133-141.

Rao, P. V., & Platt, D. E. (2008). *Effects of castor oil on wound healing and its use as a dressing.* Pharmacognosy Magazine, 4(16), 293-296.

Salunkhe, D. K., & Desai, B. B. (2010*). Postharvest biotechnology of castor oil: A critical analysis. Critical Reviews in Biotechnology,* 30(2), 1-19.

Silva, J. P., & Almeida, T. (2012). *Castor oil in cosmetic and therapeutic applications. International Journal of Cosmetic Science,* 34(1), 13-20.

Tahmassebi, J. F., & Curzon, M. E. J. (2003). *The therapeutic properties of castor oil and its historical use in various cultures.* Journal of Ethnopharmacology, 87(2-3), 135-137.